DATE DUE

JUN 2 6 2019	

MUDRAS

OF

INDIA

of related interest

The Healing Power of Mudras
The Yoga of the Hands
Rajendar Menen
ISBN 978 1 84819 043 6
eISBN 978 0 85701 024 7

Chinese Shamanic Cosmic Orbit Qigong
Esoteric Talismans, Mantras, and Mudras in Healing and Inner Cultivation
Master Zhongxian Wu
ISBN 978 1 84819 056 6
eISBN 978 0 85701 059 9

MUDRAS

OF

INDIA

A Comprehensive Guide to the Hand
Gestures of Yoga and Indian Dance

CAIN CARROLL AND REVITAL CARROLL

FOREWORD BY DR. DAVID FRAWLEY

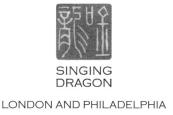

SINGING
DRAGON

LONDON AND PHILADELPHIA

First published in 2012
by Singing Dragon
an imprint of Jessica Kingsley Publishers
116 Pentonville Road
London N1 9JB, UK
and
400 Market Street, Suite 400
Philadelphia, PA 19106, USA

www.singingdragon.com

Library of Congress Cataloging in Publication Data
Carroll, Cain.
  Mudras of India : a comprehensive guide to the hand gestures of yoga and Indian dance / Cain Carroll
and Revital Carroll.
    pages cm
  Includes bibliographical references and index.
  ISBN 978-1-84819-084-9 (alk. paper)
  1. Mudras (Hinduism) 2. Yoga. 3. Gesture in dance--India. I. Carroll, Revital. II. Title.
  BL1226.82.M93C37 2012
  294.5'37--dc23
                              2012002726

British Library Cataloguing in Publication Data
A CIP catalogue record for this book is available from the British Library

ISBN 978 1 84819 084 9
eISBN 978 0 85701 067 4

Printed and bound in Great Britain

For Yashodhara Enz
Always follow your heart

CONTENTS

FOREWORD

Hand mudras or hand gestures have an important role in yogic thought and Indian culture, where they have probably been explained in more detail than perhaps any other tradition. Yet this knowledge can be helpful to all of us in bringing more meaning into our awareness and into our expression. The hands are the focus of most of what we do, reflecting how we relate to life and how we touch the world. When our energy is strong, clear, and creative in the hands, our vitality and attention, are similarly energized and directed in a positive manner. When there is no focus or attention in our hands, our lives also often lack focus and proper motivation.

Hand mudras have three main places of traditional usage in India, which are all covered in the present detailed book. The first, and most commonly known in the West, is in yoga practice, to channel higher energies into the body and mind. Mudras play a role along with asanas, pranayama, mantra and meditation in Raja Yoga and Hatha Yoga, and are becoming part of regular yoga classes.

The second place for mudras is in ritual, in which various gestures relate to different deities or their powers. Most Hindu and Buddhist rituals employ mudras as an integral part of their practice, along with special mantras and offerings. Such rituals can be part of yoga practice as well, particularly in devotional practices. In this way, mudras are not simply a means of personal expression or self-empowerment, but ways of communicating with the deity, often in meditation, and drawing divine grace in our lives.

The third is in Indian dance and drama, in which mudras reflect various types of meaning and have a symbolic value, particularly for projecting certain attitudes and emotions, or representing various powers or deities. Mudras are part of an artistic language of poetry, gesture, and dance and aid in a deeper self-expression and creative unfoldment.

The hands are our seat of pranic connection and expansion in Ayurvedic medicine, and much of healing is through the hands. Mudras can help direct higher pranic energies into the body and link us with beneficial pranic currents in nature and in the universe as a whole. Mudras relate to the marmas and nadis, the energy points and currents in the physical and subtle bodies. This can afford them tremendous healing powers and the ability to change how our energy moves and works. Mudras can be brought into various types of massage and bodywork for great benefit.

Mudras can be used along with pranayama in order to direct the prana in various ways, both internally and externally, whether to different parts of our own bodies or to the pranic fields of other people. In fact, the more power of prana one has, the greater the power one can direct through mudras. The mudra forms a vehicle for one's prana, and helps both activate and exercise the prana that one has. One can heal through mudras alone, either as directed by the practitioner or as practiced by the patient.

Mudras, especially those of the hand, are prominent in the Tantric aspect of the greater yoga tradition, and are sometimes regarded as an entire branch of practice, like asana, pranayama, mantra, or yantra. Mudras are often used along with different asanas, particularly sitting poses, where they have specific powers to energize the asanas at a deeper level.

Mudras can also serve to focus the mind and direct its power of attention. As such, mudras help prepare the mind for meditation and can reinforce certain meditational attitudes. Hand mudras can be seen like hand mantras as ways of energizing our expression. They can be used like yantras or geometrical devises for organizing our subtle energy patterns. Certain mudras are used for teachers while teaching students to focus the power of the mind, as teaching gestures. The mudra itself can project the knowledge and awareness of the teacher, like the famous Chin Mudra or "gesture of consciousness."

Mudras of India by Cain and Revital Carroll is a well-referenced guide to mudra practice, with numerous quotes from important traditional Sanskrit sources and yoga texts. It covers the full diversity of approaches to mudras found in the various spiritual traditions of India. It clearly explains how to perform particular mudras, with ease and clarity, and outlines their various levels of application, including their yogic and healing usages. The book covers all aspects of mudra practice with depth, simplicity, and precision. It is also quite detailed and lists a large number of mudras, including the most important ones commonly used, perhaps more than any other available publication.

Mudras of India is an important handbook for mudra practice, helpful to any yoga or health practitioner. It is well-illustrated and very practical in its design, making it useful for a wide variety of students and scholars. It is probably the most detailed book on the subject in the English language and the best organized, making the science of mudra accessible to everyone. There have been a number of books on mudras done in recent years, of varying degrees of value. However, if there is a single book on mudra that one could recommend, I would recommend this book to start with.

Dr. David Frawley
Director, American Institute of Vedic Studies (www.vedanet.com)
Author of Yoga and Ayurveda *and* Yoga for Your Type

ACKNOWLEDGMENTS

We are grateful to all the yogis and dancers who have carried forth the rich tradition of hand mudras throughout the centuries, and to all of the talented and inspiring people who helped us bring this project to fruition. Thank you to Reed Rahn for his magic with the camera during our Phoenix photo shoots, to Phil Timper for all his work rendering the mudra images (and Nancy Timper for not breaking the bank), to Dilip Kumar Dhirsamant for his endurance and patience during our long photo shoot in Bhubaneswar, to Sanskrit scholar, Nicolai Bachman, for his editorial suggestions and rendering of the Devanagari and transliteration of the mudra names, to Dr. Mandakranta Bose for her wise counsel and editorial suggestions, and to our publisher, Jessica Kingsley, for her sincere interest in seeing this book come to life, and the whole team at Singing Dragon for their patience, flexibility, and professionalism.

From Cain

I am deeply grateful to all of my teachers, and the generations of lineage masters who came before, who have inspired and informed my practice of mudras and the many other dimensions of internal cultivation: Baba Hari Das, Satjivan Singh, Ari Singh, Yogi Das, Dr. Yogi Vikeshanand, Banambar Baba, Master Zhongxian Wu, Liu Shan, Daoist Yogi Ramkohea, Dr. Matt Schlechten, and Sun Yogi Umashankar. I offer my heartfelt gratitude to all of my family and friends who lift me up with their unending support, to my friend and colleague, Laraine Herring, for all her helpful writing tips, playful encouragement, and mostly for being a living example of a "writing warrior," and to all of my students who continue to inspire me with their sincere desire to learn and practice the yogic arts. Special thanks to my loving wife and coauthor, Revital Carroll, for being my trusted partner in this book project and in our everyday life together.

From Revital

I extend my heartfelt gratitude to all my teachers who took the time to share their vast knowledge of hand mudras with me. I extend special thanks to my first Odissi Dance teacher, the late Guru Gangadhar Pradhan, and his senior disciple Sri Lingaraj Swain, for initially introducing me to the art of dance mudras and their proper usage, and for instilling in me the passion to always aspire to expand my knowledge and remain an eternal student. My deepest gratitude goes to Guru Bichitrananda Swain and Sri Pabhitra Kumar Pradhan for their willingness to engage in conversation about the subtle meanings of the numerous mudras applications. I am grateful to my dance teachers: Sri Yudishtir Nayak, Smt. Sujata Mohapatra, Guru Rathikant Mohapatra, and Smt. Niharika Mohanty, from whom I am continuously learning more about the form, grace, and proper usage of hand mudras in Classical Indian Dance. I am filled with infinite appreciation to Guru Kelucharan Mohapatra, whom I never had the grace of meeting in person, but who influences my dance journey multifold through all of my teachers, and through the Odissi Research Institute, with its immense contribution to the study of hand gestures. I thank all of my yoga and meditation teachers for stoking the fire of spiritual aspiration within me, and for continuing to inspire me to follow my intuition, passion, and devotion as I deepen my practice. My special thanks to Clive Sheridan, my first teacher of Tantric hand mudras, whom I met while wandering through India in the early 1990s. I offer my sincere appreciation to Kali Ray for sharing her unique and inspirational relationship with the practice of hand mudras, and intriguing me to deepen my intuitive relation to the power in my hands. I thank all of my students, colleagues, and friends for encouraging and inspiring me to continue to learn and share my knowledge with them. And last but not least, I thank my husband, Cain Carroll, for his vision, unwavering support and encouragement, and for believing in me.

SANSKRIT PRONUNCIATION GUIDE

Standard Academic Transliteration

In an effort to uphold the rich tradition of Sanskrit as the language of yoga and Indian dance, we have selected to render the names of each mudra in English, Devanagari, and Transliteration (English with standard academic diacritical markings). For the convenience of the lay reader we have chosen to separate many of the longer Sanskrit names and titles into separate words for easier readability. For example, Abhayahṛdayamudrā becomes Abhaya Hrdaya Mudra, with the latter being the standard way we reference the mudra throughout the text. Most Sanskrit words in the body of the text are italicized, immediately followed by the word's literal English translation in parentheses and quotation marks.

Vowels

a	another
ā	father (2 beats)
i	pin
ī	need (2 beats)
u	flute
ū	mood (2 beats)
ṛ	macabre
e	etude (2 beats)
ai	aisle (2 beats)
o	yoke (2 beats)
au	flautist (2 beats)

Special Letters

aṁ   h<u>um</u>

aḥ   out-breath

Consonants

ka   papri<u>k</u>a

kha   thi<u>ck h</u>oney

ga   sa<u>g</u>a

gha   bi<u>g h</u>oney

ṅa   i<u>n</u>k

ca   <u>ch</u>utney

cha   mu<u>ch h</u>oney

ja   Japan

jha   ra<u>j h</u>oney

ña   i<u>n</u>ch

ṭa   borsch<u>t</u> again

ṭha   borsch<u>t h</u>oney

ḍa   sh<u>d</u>um

ḍha   sh<u>d h</u>um

ṇa   sh<u>n</u>um

ta   pas<u>t</u>a

tha   ea<u>t h</u>oney

da   so<u>d</u>a

dha   goo<u>d h</u>oney

na   bana<u>n</u>a

pa   <u>p</u>aternal

pha   scoo<u>p h</u>oney

ba   scu<u>b</u>a

bha	ru<u>b h</u>oney
ma	aro<u>m</u>a
ya	emplo<u>y</u>able
ra	abra cadab<u>r</u>a
la	hu<u>l</u>a
va	<u>v</u>ariety
śa	<u>sh</u>ut
ṣa	<u>sch</u>napps
sa	Li<u>s</u>a
ha	<u>h</u>oney

In Sanskrit, when two vowels meet they will combine into something else. For example, "dhātu" plus "agni" becomes "dhātvagni" and "bhūta" plus "agni" becomes "bhūtāgni."

Some Sanskrit sounds are pronounced slightly differently in North and South India. The "v" might sound like a "w" and the "ś" or "ṣ" may sound like a "sh" or a "s."

There are some differences between Sanskrit and Hindi pronunciation. In Sanskrit, when a word ends with an "a" it is pronounced. In Hindi it is often dropped, even though it is written the same way. For example, the Sanskrit "Āyurveda" sounds like "Āyurved" in Hindi.

Sanskrit	**Hindi**
"a" at the end of a word is pronounced	"a" at the end of a word is often not pronounced
"ā" at the end of a word is long	"ā" at the end of a word is pronounced as short "a"
"ph" pronounced as an aspirated "p"	"ph" can also be pronounced like "f"

NOTE Sanskrit Pronunciation Guide used with permission from Nicolai Bachman at www.sanskritsounds.com.

INTRODUCTION

The History and Heritage of Mudras

The hands are a source of tremendous power. With such profound dexterity, sensitivity, and utility, the human hands may be one of our most defining features as a species. Playing guitar, delivering a baby, knitting a sweater, building a house, wielding a sword, painting intricate figures: through the use of our hands we create and shape the world we live in. Hands can heal, hands can harm. One touch can convey a wide array of thoughts, feelings, or intentions. Hands tell the story of our mood or state of mind. When we feel angry, a clenched fist; when anxious, fidgeting fingers. Even plants and animals respond to the subtle nuances of our touch.

With the hands playing such a central role in our experience of being human, it comes as no surprise that many of the world's great spiritual and artistic traditions have considered the hands as sacred. With five digits, twenty-seven bones, and fifteen joints—plus numerous carpal joints affording articulation of the wrist—the human hand is a masterpiece of nature. Perhaps, this is why many cultures throughout history viewed the human hand as a perfect microcosm of the universe. For example, the shaman kings (*Wu*) of ancient China viewed all things in the animated world as emanations of the changing relationship between five fundamental principles (commonly referred to as the Five Elements): Water, Wood, Fire, Earth, and Metal. They viewed the human hand as one of the most poignant examples of these five principles, with each of the fingers representing one the Five Elements (Earth/thumb, Metal/index, Water/little, Wood/ring, and Fire/middle). These relationships, and the character of each finger based on the theory of Five Elements, are woven into the philosophy and practice of all the traditional Chinese arts: calligraphy, Traditional Chinese Medicine, astrology, martial arts, *cha dao* (tea culture), classical music, dance, and theater.

In many of these arts, specific hand positions and gestures are used in relationship to the precise effect desired by the practitioner. For example, a Chinese shaman might instruct a patient suffering from anxiety to tuck her thumbs into her palms and hold them firmly. Since the thumb relates to Earth, closing the other fingers around it creates an energetic seal, a mudra, which imparts a sense of safety and stability, thus reducing anxiety. In Chinese calligraphy, the brush is held firmly with the thumb, index, middle, and ring finger while the little finger is tucked slightly in and not used. This is in an effort to conserve the energy of the kidneys (Water), giving the calligrapher a certain vitality that can be seen in the *qi* of their brush strokes.

A similar tradition emerged in ancient India, where Vedic sages and Tantric yogis developed a highly nuanced cosmology with the *Pancha Maha Bhuta* ("Five Great Elements") as the basic foundation. The *Pancha Maha Bhuta* of the Indian cosmological system is similar, but not identical to, the Five Element theory used throughout East Asia.

Pancha Maha Bhuta

Element (English)	Element (Sanskrit)
Fire	*Agni*
Air	*Vayu*
Ether/Space	*Akasha*
Earth	*Prithivi*
Water	*Apas*

Indian *rishis* (seers) discovered a direct connection between the *Pancha Maha Bhuta* and the five fingers of the human hand. They emphasized that the relationship of the *Pancha Maha Bhuta* in the body should remain balanced and in harmony with the rest of the natural world. They taught that any disorder in the body or mind indicates an excess or deficiency in one or more of the Elements. Through centuries of research and experimentation with techniques used to influence the *bhutas*—as well as influential exchanges with other Asian traditions—they developed an elaborate system called *Yoga Tattva Mudra Vijnana*.[1] This unique branch of Vedic wisdom clearly describes the relationship between the five fingers and Five Elements, and sets forth an extensive system of mudras whose influence is seen in many of the classical disciplines of India: dance, theater, architecture, painting, medicine (*Ayurveda*), martial arts, and yoga. Since all the classical arts of India were evolving within the context of Vedic and Tantric spirituality, the cosmology of the *Pancha Maha Bhuta* and the presence of mudras are almost ubiquitous.

The Sanskrit word *mudra* means "attitude," "gesture," or "seal." The most common use of the word describes the many hand gestures used in yoga, spiritual ritual, and Indian dance. It is these hand gestures (*hasta mudras*) that are the main focus of this book. However, it is important to understand that *mudra* has many other meanings used in numerous different contexts. For example, the *Kularnava Tantra*[2] traces the word *mudra* to the root *mud* ("to delight in") and *dru* ("to give" or "draw forth"). This hints at an ecstatic state of non-duality, or union with the deity, as the ultimate definition of *mudra*. In the *Siva Sutras*, one of the most important texts of Kashmir Shaivism, *mudra* is mentioned in two contexts: as *mudra-virya* and *mudra-krama*. *Mudra-virya* refers to the underlying power that reveals the ground of our experience as *Turya* ("pure awareness").[3] *Mudra-krama* is a densely loaded phrase that connotes the state in which the mind alternates between internal awareness of "self" and external awareness of "the world," and thus cannot find a true distinction between the two. Due to this power called *samavesha* ("co-existence"), the practitioner's consciousness is perfectly merged with the way things are. In this context, *mudra* is the sense of having united with something larger, while simultaneously knowing that such a union is primordial.

The word *mudra* also refers to the large earrings worn by Kanphata Yogis[4] in India, an order of *sadhus* (religious ascetics) who follow the teachings of Gorakhnath (a famous Nath Yogi and prolific author who lived in the tenth or eleventh century). In Indian Tantrism, *mudra* is also used to denote the parched grains used in Tantric ritual, and also as a subtle reference to the female consort, called *Shakti* or *Dakini*, of a Tantric yogin. The Kagyu sect of *Vajrayana* Buddhism uses the suffix *maha* ("great") in conjunction with the term *mudra* to describe the lineage's quintessential meditation practice called *Mahamudra* ("the Great Seal"). In this context, the word *mudra* refers the a specific method of meditation and its fruition. *Mahamudra* describes the practice of looking directly at the fundamental nature of Mind. It also denotes the highest enlightenment, where Mind and Emptiness are synonymous.[5]

Mudras in the Yoga Tradition

In the Hatha Yoga tradition, mudras are considered precious tools on the path of awakening. There are five classes of such mudras taught in the yoga tradition: *hasta* ("hand"), *mana* ("head"), *kaya* ("postural"), *bandha* ("lock"), and *adhara* ("base") or ("perineal"). Although these five are different, they share the common purpose of serving as "seals" or "locks" used to affect the flow of energy in particular organs and channels of the body. The *Gheranda Samhita* (a seventeenth-century text on Hatha Yoga) describes twenty-five of these types of mudras.[6] Each of the five classes of mudras contains numerous techniques used for different purposes. Many of the postural mudras and locks form the basis for the internal practices of Hatha Yoga that—contrary to the popular application of yoga as a fitness fad—are aimed primarily at affecting the autonomic nervous system, and have very little to do with the appearance of the musculoskeletal system.

Hasta Mudra is the name given to the many hand gestures, such as *Surabhi Mudra* (see p.243), used in Hatha Yoga to regulate the flow of *prana* ("life force") and ready the mind for meditation. The *Soma Shambhu Paddhati* (circa tenth century) describes thirty-seven hand mudras, the most common being *Abhaya Mudra, Anjali Mudra, Chin Mudra, Dhyana Mudra,* and *Jnana Mudra. Mana Mudras* work with the "seven openings" of the head (two eyes, two ears, two nostrils, and mouth). With practices such as *Shanmukha Mudra* (see p.222), the various *Mana Mudras* are used mainly as techniques of *pratyahara* ("internalization of the senses") to systematically direct consciousness inward toward the object of meditation. *Kaya Mudras* such as *Vipareetakarni* are bodily postures (*asanas*) combined with specific breathing techniques and visualizations. They are most commonly used to open *chakras* ("energy centers") and awaken *Kundalini* ("serpent power"). *Bandha Mudras* such as *Maha Vedha Mudra* employ *bandhas* ("interior locks") along with *asanas* ("postures") and *kumbhaka* ("breath retention"). These are used for similar purposes as the *Kaya Mudras*, and are often found sequenced together in traditional sets of practice. *Adhara Mudras* such as *Ashvini Mudra* utilize various methods of contracting the musculature of the anus, sexual organs, and perineum to stimulate the endocrine system and strengthen the body's vital energy.

According to the doctrine of *Yoga Tattva Mudra Vijnana*, all diseases in the body and disturbances of mind result from the imbalance of the Five Elements and disruption of the natural flow of *prana*. Through centuries of use and refinement, the techniques of the five classes of mudras have been shown to be a highly effective system of self-healing and spiritual cultivation. The passage below conveys the supreme importance of mudras in the yoga tradition:

> Therefore, the goddess sleeping at the entrance of *Brahma's* door should be constantly aroused with all effort by performing mudras thoroughly. *Maha Mudra, Maha Bandha, Maha Vedha, Khechari, Uddiyana, Mula Bandha, Jalandhara Bandha, Viparita Karani Mudra, Vajroli,* and *Shakti Chalana,* verily, these are the ten mudras which destroy old age and death. *Adinath*[7] said they are the bestowers of the eight powers. They are held in high esteem by all the *siddhas* [adepts] and are difficult for even gods to attain. These must remain secret like precious stones, and not be talked about to anybody... (Hatha Yoga Pradipika, chapter 3, verses 5–9)[8]

Of the five classes of mudras, *Hasta Mudras* are the most numerous and widely used throughout India. Compared with the other four classes of mudras—many of which require direct instruction from a competent teacher—most hand mudras are easy to learn and safe to practice on your own. Following common sense, intuitive guidance, and some diligent practice, hand mudras can serve as side-effect-free health care, first aid in the case of acute illness, natural treatment of chronic illness or injury, and as a do-it-yourself method of developing latent psycho-energetic potential. For example, *Mritsamjivani Mudra* (see p.159) is traditionally used in the case of acute heart attack, and is affectionately called the "lifesaving mudra." *Apana Mudra* (see p.45) is used to assist the ease of delivery when a woman is in labor, and can also be use daily to treat chronic constipation. For yoga students and teachers, the use of hand mudras such as *Prana Mudra* (see p.193) during asana practice can greatly enhance the energetic effects of poses, as well as the mental, emotional, and spiritual benefits of the practice.

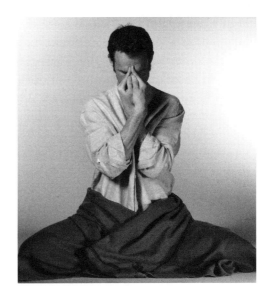

NIRVANA MUDRA

Hand mudras can be classified into four basic groups: (1) those held by deities or used in the iconographic depictions of gods, demigods, demons, or heroes of epic stories such as the *Mahabharata*; (2) those used in rites, rituals, and Tantric worship, such as *japa* ("repetition of prayers"), *avahana* ("invocations"), *kamya-karma* ("rites of abundance"), *naivedya* ("offering food"), and *snana* ("bathing"); (3) those used in yogic practices for concentration, energy cultivation, healing, or evoking desired states of consciousness; and (4) those used in performance arts, such as dance and theater, for story telling and emotional expression. The four groups of hand mudras can be further divided into two sub-groups: *asamyukta hastas* ("single-hand gestures") and *samyukta hastas* ("joint-hand gestures"). There is also a long tradition in India, mostly among esoteric yogis, of mudras occurring spontaneously during deep meditation. This unfolds through a phenomenon called *prana vidya* ("direct cognition of energy"), where the yogi expresses subtle internal states through unprompted gestures and movements.

> "Mudra means 'seal', and the mudras are concerned with the mind. Practicing the mudras keeps the mind fixed on the points over which they are applied." (Swami Satchidananda)[9]

Mudras are used in the religious, spiritual, and artistic traditions of many cultures throughout the world. The emblem of the Jain religion is called the "Jain Hand," an iconic depiction of *Abhaya Mudra* with images of a *dharmachakra* ("wheel of dharma") and the word *ahimsa* ("non-violence") in the center of the palm.

Mudras are common in Jain symbolism and mentioned in spiritual literature such as the *Bhairav Padmavati Kalp*.

Tantric gestures are commonly seen in Bhutan, Tibet, Nepal, China, and Japan. Ritual mudras and meditation gestures are seen in Burma, Vietnam, Thailand, and Laos. Dramatic mudras are seen in the dance and theater traditions of India, Nepal, Thailand, Sri Lanka, and Bali. In iconographic images of Jesus Christ giving benediction, he is often seen with his right hand in a specific gesture—not unlike *Prana Mudra* (see p.193) in yoga or *Ardhapataka Mudra* (see p.50) in dance —where the thumb, index, and middle fingers are extended upward, and the ring and little bent toward the palm. Mother Mary is frequently depicted with her hands to her sides, palms facing forward and slightly up

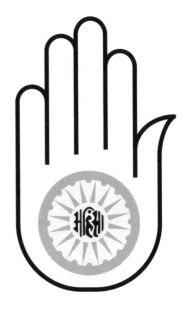

JAIN HAND

in a receptive position. This gesture evokes a similar sentiment of bestowing blessings as *Varada Mudra* (see p.266), commonly seen in Southeast Asian depictions of the Buddha.

Throughout the Middle East and North Africa, the *Hamsa* is used as an amulet and universal sign of protection. The Arabic word *hamsa* literally means "five." The emblem relates to the five senses, the five daily prayers, and hints at the idea of "five fingers in the eye of evil," a cultural reference to the perceived power generated by specific hand positions. The *Hamsa* emblem of a downward-facing right hand is the source of profound symbolism for numerous religious groups. It is called the "Hand of Miriam" by the Jewish, the "Hand of Fatima" by Muslims, and the "Hand of Mary" by Christians. It is interesting to note that the *Hamsa* represents a feminine quality across traditions. Worn on the body as jewelry, or placed on a door or window, it serves a similar purpose of dispelling fear, granting good fortune, and repelling negative energies as *Abhaya Mudra* (see p.34) in Hindu and Buddhist traditions.

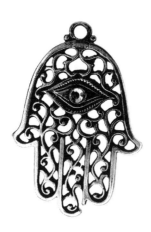

HAMSA

Mudras in Classical Indian Dance

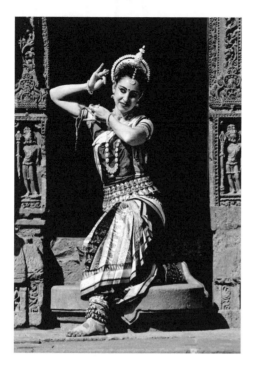

ODISSI DANCER AT RAJARANI
TEMPLE

In Classical Indian Dance there is a significant emphasis on the conscious formation of hand gestures. The hands are always held in an intentional manner and in a definite mudra. The ground for such a unique feature in a dance form lies in the cultural context it emerged within. Indian dance was developed side by side with the spiritual–religious philosophy of the subcontinent, valuing the potentiality in our hands to generate and direct energy. The prominent role hand gestures play in Indian dance strongly links them to the other arts and spiritual traditions of India.

Mudras are used in Classical Indian Dance for story telling and expressing the subtleties of human emotion and relationship. Similar to the yoga tradition, they are also used following the view of Tantra, for the purposes of transformation and evolution by stimulating the flow of *shakti* ("primal force") in the organs, glands, and nerve channels of the body.

A clear understanding of how hand gestures are used in Indian dance would not be possible without a basic familiarity with the origin and scope of practice of Classical Indian Dance as a whole. Dance has been an important component of Indian society for millennia, and it is associated as a form of expression and celebration of all the significant moments of human life: birth, death, courtship, marriage, victory, defeat, and so on. It is utilized as a form of spiritual and devotional practice, a medium for communication and communion with the Divine, and as a channel to carry forth the spiritual and religious teachings of an era. While the feet form a stable foundation and set the rhythm of the dance, the hands—being at the end of the creative channels (*nadis*) of the arms—are the most potent body part to convey the expressional aspect of the dance/drama tradition.

The ancient texts on drama and dance refer to hand gestures as *hastas*, whereas the term *mudra* has historically denoted hand gestures connected with religious ritual. In the recent past, since Classical Indian Dance was revived in the earlier part of the twentieth century, we find that the term *hasta* is no longer widely used to describe hand gestures by practicing dancers. The general term *mudra* is now commonly used by both dancers and spiritual practitioners. Although *hasta* is technically the correct term for dance hand gestures, we have chosen to use *mudra* in reference to all gestures since it is the more broadly known term.

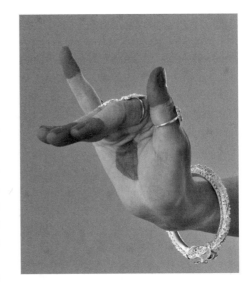

MRIGASHIRSHA MUDRA

Many dance traditions have emerged throughout India, each with its own regional texts. However, the earliest and most influential of all texts on dance is the *Natya Shastra*. It is generally believed to have been written between 200 BCE and 200 CE by Bharata Muni, and is considered the original treatise on music, dance, and theatre. According to the *Natya Shashtra*, the four forms of *abhinaya* ("expression") in Indian dance and drama are classified as:

1. *Vachika*—verbal (song)

2. *Angika*—bodily, mainly mudras

3. *Aharya*—costume and makeup

4. *Satvika*—mood and sentiment, mainly expressed through the face.

A number of other texts follow closely after the *Natya Shastra*. Among them is the *Abhinaya Darpana* of Nandikeshvara, the first practical text solely devoted to dance. This is perhaps the most influential text in the field of dance technique, and extensively deals with the use of hand gestures for communication and expression. As such, we have chosen to follow the variations of hand mudras listed in the *Abhinaya Darpana*, while using the *Natya Shastra* as a secondary resource. Over the centuries, primarily from the thirteenth century onwards, many regions in India developed their own manuals of dance and unique technique that vary slightly from the standard versions of the mudras. In the spirit of thoroughness, we have included some of these commonly used mudras from regional texts. However, it would be overwhelming and confusing to try to include them all, since often they are almost identical to the original texts with slight variations or name changes.

Classical Indian Dance technique is generally divided into *nritta* (pure technical dance, that does not express any particular mood or conveys a narrative), and *nritya* (expressive dance, accompanying the unfolding of a story and meaning of song lyrics). *Natya* is yet another category mentioned in the *Natya Shastra* and other treatises, and it exclusively corresponds to drama. The vast majority of dance mudras have a versatile scope of usage and are employed in context of *nritya* ("expression") as well as *nritta* ("pure dance"). Some of the dance mudras are exclusively of the *nritya* category and are solely used for specific applications of expression. In the model of Classical Indian Dance, the hands are the only body part that possess both *nritta* and *nritya* qualities. The face (eyebrows, eyes, eyelids, nose, lips, etc.)

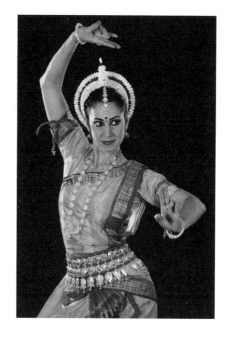

ODISSI DANCER (MAYURA MUDRA)

is primarily used for expression, while the feet, legs, waist, and chest carry out the technical movement.

Classical Indian Dance technique views the joints as the initiators of movement, and shapers of form. Therefore, in Indian dance, rather than initiating movement from the muscles of the hands or arms, every mudra is articulated and initiated from the wrist. This change of focus imbues each mudra with a certain connectivity that carries the impact of the gesture deep into the dancer's core and the spectator's heart. Each mudra carries numerous possibilities of movement and is a portal for an entire language of animated gesticulation. The mudras in dance are the focal point around which everything else revolves. The verse below, from the *Abhinaya Darpana*, poetically describes the importance of *mudras*:

> *Yato hastas tato drishtih*
> *Yato drishitis tato manah*
> *Yato manas tato bhavo*
> *Yato bhavas tato rasah.*[10]

> "Where the hand goes, the eyes follow.
> Where the eyes go, the mind follows.
> Where the mind (awareness) is, mood or emotion (*bhava*) is
>   created.
> Once *bhava* is created, sentiment (*rasa*) arises."

This verse also illustrates the central role of emotional expression in Indian dance. The intention of evoking sentiment in the viewer, largely through the use of mudras and facial expression, is built into the structure and technique of classical dance and is seen as a path to spiritual awakening. Unfortunately, many of the subtle energetics and spiritual implications of mudras in dance have been forgotten over the centuries. Dancers are often taught a complete repertoire of mudras, along with the corresponding movements and rhythmic steps, without learning the deeper spiritual heritage behind these.

The same is true in the modern expression of yoga, where spiritually stylized fitness has taken the popular spotlight over the traditional more contemplative side of the practice. In modern times, we often see beautiful mudras being performed merely for the sake of aesthetics. Although such performances can be interesting for the eye, they fail to touch the more profound experience that is possible when the spiritual power behind mudras is accessed. The importance of the subtle inner workings of mudras, not only their outward appearance, is a value shared by yoga and Indian dance alike. It is for this reason that we have chosen to include the mudras of both dance and yoga in one book.

Although yoga and Indian dance share the same heritage and spiritual values, they are distinct traditions, each with its own repository of mudras. In their classical application, mudras from dance often do not cross over to yoga, and vice versa. However, we feel strongly that each tradition has tremendous value to offer the other. Practitioners of yoga and meditation can greatly enhance their *sadhana* ("practice") by learning the art of emotional expression implicit in the use of dance mudras. The emphasis placed on rousing the sentiments of the heart is a central theme in both dance and *Bhakti Yoga* ("path of devotion"). We have found that this important component of spiritual life is greatly enriched by working with the theatrical mudras and *rasas* ("moods") used in dance. Similarly, incorporating yoga mudras into their daily training, dancers will be guided to connect with the spiritual power inherent in the ancient roots of the dance. The meditative practice of yoga mudras will improve a dancer's overall health, increase mental clarity, and develop superior concentration for learning complex choreography.

The creative capacity contained in the hands is accessible to anyone. Whether you are a dancer, yogi/yogini, spiritual seeker, or simply feel drawn to explore something new, the realm of hand mudras has much to offer. We hope you will enjoy this simple and powerful way to access your core being, nurture body and mind, and bring an added element of beauty and devotion to your life.

Getting Started

For many years we have nurtured a deep interest in the beauty and power of hand mudras. We find great joy in practicing the mudras presented here and we are delighted to share this information with you. Our desire in presenting this material is two-fold: (1) to provide an easy-to-reference encyclopedic guide to the large body of mudras used in the Indian tradition; (2) to provide a practical resource to inform and inspire readers to take up a personal practice of hand mudras. We have endeavored to include the most widely used mudras of India. However, the tradition of hand mudras in India is extremely vast, with numerous regional texts in local dialects, as well as many oral traditions that teach seemingly endless variations of mudras. Different schools and styles of dance and yoga use different hand gestures and different terms for the same mudras. Most systems, however, share a similar set of names and applications that is congruent with the information in this book. Where applicable, we have included alternate names for the mudras to help you cross-reference gestures between traditions. Below are some things to consider as you continue your journey into the fascinating realm of hand mudras.

About the Book Format

The mudras are listed A to Z by their Sanskrit name rendered in English. Below the main listing you will see the name again in Devanagari (Sanskrit script), and once more in English with academic transliteration markings to assist in correct pronunciation of the original Sanskrit. Next to each mudra listing you will see a small icon:

means this mudra has a spiritual/religious context and it is found in one or many of the spiritual traditions that developed in India.

means this mudra is found in texts and sources related to the dance and drama traditions of India.

Occasionally, a mudra is shared by both traditions and will be indicated by the presence of both icons.

You will notice some mudras have benefits listed, others do not. Since many of the dance mudras are used in the context of performing, story telling, and expression (*abhinaya*) they do not traditionally have associated benefits, per se. In some cases, where we have personally experienced healing benefits of a specific dance mudra, we have taken the liberty of including a short list of such benefits based on our own experience and knowledge of the *Yoga Tattva Mudra Vijnana*.

General Tips on Practicing Mudras

The underlying power of mudras exists in feeling the subtle energetic effects in your own body. Whether you are practicing yoga mudras for healing or spiritual cultivation, or dance mudras for emotional and aesthetic expression, the secret to taking your experience deeper is to slow down, concentrate on the subtleties of each gesture, and really feel the effects of what you are doing. Practicing single-hand (*asamyukta*) mudras with each hand will increase the benefits. However, if a mudra cannot be made with each hand, there is still great benefit in practicing with one hand. This is especially true in the case of injury or disease in one hand, or even the loss of a hand or arm.

The hands in their basic resting form—open and relaxed—represent the realm of pure potential. This potential is neutral. You can select what you want to manifest by performing any number of mudras after taking a moment of stillness with the hands in their natural position. Practicing this way, you activate what is always present in the formless state. If you are new to mudras, you can practice three to four mudras at a time to create a balanced set based on your specific focus. If you are familiar with the practice of hand gestures, you can string together as many mudras as you like. There is no hard rule as to the order of mudras practiced. We encourage you to experiment, using your own intuition and sensitivity as your guide. Further information on sequences and traditional sets of mudras can be found in the Appendices.

Aside from the holistic benefits of mudras, working with hand gestures is also wonderful for the health of the hands themselves. For the physical benefit of the joints, tendons, ligaments, and cartilage of the hands, it is good to extend the fingers vigorously and activate your muscular strength while holding the mudras. To stimulate the more subtle energetic effects, and to affect the whole body and mind through the Five Element finger relationships, it is better to keep the hands soft and relaxed while performing mudras. We generally recommend incorporating both methods of practice in a given session, or alternating methods each day you practice. In this way, you maximize both the physical and psycho-spiritual benefits of your practice.

Here are a few more general recommendations:

1. Be gentle with your fingers. Some of the mudras may challenge the flexibility of your finger joints, and it is not uncommon to feel a little sore

after practicing some of the more complex mudras. If you have arthritis in your hands, practicing mudras is especially helpful, yet even more caution and gentleness needs to be employed.

2. Do not practice on a full stomach.

3. Use your mind to send energy into your hands, and become aware of each and every finger and part of your hands, wrists, and your entire body. Activating the energy in your hands will in turn activate the corresponding energy in your body and will make your entire being feel more alive and awake.

4. While practicing the various hand gestures, articulate the precise form as described in this text to the best of your ability, while bearing in mind that we all have slightly different body proportions, and our anatomical differences will reflect in the subtle variations of our hand gestures.

Warming up the Hands

Since performing mudras is like a yoga session for your hands, it is good to take a little time to warm up the fingers before beginning to work with the mudras. Here is a simple warm-up that just takes a moment. Take a deep breath in and hold your breath. Clap the hands together firmly three times, hard enough so that they sting just a little bit. Exhale slowly through the mouth and resume natural breathing. Then, rub the hands together vigorously for about one minute, or until they feel very warm. Make sure to rub the palms and tops of the hands and fingers, warming the hands on all sides, even between the fingers. This easy warm-up will improve blood circulation to the hands and fingers, make the joints feel more supple and strong, and increase your sensitivity to the energy generated through your mudra practice.

Tips on Practicing Yoga Mudras

Traditionally, yogic mudras used for healing and spiritual cultivation are practiced while seated in a meditation posture, such as *padmasana* (lotus pose)[1] or *siddhasana* (adept's pose).[2] These postures, as well as the use of a meditation bench or sturdy chair, can greatly enhance your mudra practice. It is important to always maintain an erect spine, relaxed chest, and soft shoulders. This will allow your diaphragm and ribcage to move freely as you breathe. Smooth and natural breathing is what animates the mudras with life force (*prana*). Any position that inhibits your ability to breath deeply and easily should not be used for the practice of mudras. The most important thing is that you feel comfortable. Following the rules of good posture and deep breathing, mudras may be practiced just about anywhere; while walking or standing, sitting, or anytime you feel inspired. One of our favorite places for extended sessions of mudras is on long airplane flights. However, it's important to be discreet if you practice in public. Drawing attention to yourself will deter from the power of your practice. Many of the mudras may be done with your hands in your pockets, tucked under your shirt, inside mittens when it's cold out, or covered by a shawl or scarf. Practicing while traveling on planes, trains, or buses is a fun way to pass the time while strengthening your body, calming your mind, and brightening your spirit. It's like doing a full yoga practice without leaving your seat!

The Three Basic Effects of Yoga Mudras

Based on the knowledge of the *Yoga Tattva Mudra Vijnana*, there are three basic effects resulting from the practice of yoga mudras:

1. *Tonifying—The tip of the thumb touches the base of any finger.* Touching the tip of the thumb to the base of any finger will increase the Element associated with that finger. For example, touching the thumb to the base of the ring finger will strengthen the Earth Element.

2. *Sedating—Any finger covered by the thumb.* Covering any finger with the thumb causes a sedation of the Element associated with that finger. For example, covering the middle finger with the thumb, as in *Shunya Mudra* (see p.232), sedates the Ether/Space Element.

3. *Balancing—The tip of the thumb joins with the tip of any finger.* Touching the tip of the thumb to the tip of any other finger will bring the associated Element into balance with the others.

In the descriptions of the mudras in the main section, you will find occasional references to the benefits of a mudra based on its effect on the *Pancha Maha Bhuta*, *Pancha Vayu*, or Ayurvedic *dosha*. More information about these, and the Indian yogic view on energy anatomy and cosmology, can be found in Appendix A. You will also notice that many of the yoga mudras are part of a traditional set called the *Gayatri Mudras*. This is a series of twenty-four pre-meditation and eight post-meditation mudras. If you are interested in exploring a more in-depth practice incorporating this traditional set of thirty-two mudras, you can see Appendix B for the full list of *Gayatri Mudras*.

Tips on Practicing Dance Mudras

In the traditional application of dance mudras, less emphasis is placed on the healing benefits derived. Rather, it is the subtleties of creative expression that take center stage. The quality of articulating hand gestures in the context of dance includes a vital component of added movement, direction, and placement to communicate distinctive expression. We tap into the *shakti* ("primal force") within us through the conscious formation of the various hand gestures, and we utilize that creativity as we employ a specific intention.

The dance mudras included in this book are for the most part derived from the two most fundamental texts on Classical Indian Dance, the *Natya Shastra* and *Abhinaya Darapana*. These ancient treatises serve as the bedrock for all forms of Classical Indian Dance and drama. However, over the centuries, regional texts have sprung up throughout India, diverting, elaborating, and informing the numerous dance forms with their own unique language of mudra variations. It is important to recognize that dance is a living tradition that includes as many tributaries of expression as there are practitioners who carry it forth. The principal names and meanings we include in this book are those described in the *Natya Shastra* and *Abhinaya Darpana*. However, we reference mudras mentioned in the *Hasta Lakshana Deepika* (a treatise from Kerala inspiring *Katakhali* and *Mohiniyattam* usage of hand gestures), the *Abhinaya Chandrika* (see Glossary), as well as Mudras used exclusively within the Odissi Dance tradition.

You will notice *Viniyoga* (applications noted in the *Abhinaya Darapana*) terms included under many of the dance mudra's Application section. These are traditionally learned while training to become a dancer. The apprentice gains knowledge of the mudras by reciting the list of applications (*Viniyoga*) as a continuous chant, while forming the gesture with the appropriate movement and facial expression. The Sanskrit terms listed under the *Viniyoga* include the traditional endings such as "and," "with," or "etc." when appropriate. Keep in mind meanings may vary from one dance tradition to the next.

Traditionally, dance mudras are categorized into established sets and are studied as a continuous flow. The two most popular ones being the twenty-eight "single-hand mudras" (*asamyukta hasta*) and twenty-four "joint-hand mudras" (*samyukta hasta*) as described in the *Abhinaya Darpana*. These, and more of the common sets of dance mudras, are provided in Appendix C. In order to get a more in-depth familiarity with any single mudra, it is best to study the main section titled "The Mudras." However, in order to develop fluency in gesticulation, we recommend practicing the various sets in their traditional sequences.

As a rule of thumb—with some exceptions—dance hand gestures are held at least a hand's distance away from your body in order to facilitate harmonious movement in the torso and maintain connectedness in movement and grace in posture. Often, while performing, the dance gestures are held at a right angle to the arm, with the elbows lifted, arms parallel to the ground, and wrists bent. Holding the hand gestures in this manner is pleasing to the eye and arouses an unobstructed flow of creative energy to the hands and fingers.

Direct Experience is the Common Ground

Whether mudras are classified under yoga or dance, or found in various forms or sets, they all share a common ground. The essential themes found in all Vedic and Tantric arts reveal that these traditions are founded on a sincere interest in touching the heart of our humanity. In all of the great spiritual and artistic traditions of India—such as Hinduism, Buddhism, yoga, Tantra, Indian dance, drama, martial arts, etc.— one central theme emerges as paramount: How can we be free and happy? This basic human desire is the root of our shared human narrative.

Through years of exploring the potential of mudras, and sharing them with students of all walks of life, we have come to understand that each hand gesture has an intrinsic capacity to facilitate healing, concentration, creative expression, and an expansion of consciousness that is deeply rewarding. It seems that mudras hold the power to transform raw life-energy into subtle spiritual expression. This experience of spirit is unique for each of us. Inexplicable, yet undeniable, it is inherent in the way we naturally are. It is echoed in the heart's innermost yearnings. At the end of the day, only you know what that feels like. Direct experience is our common spiritual ground.

With that said, we hope you will feel inspired by the information presented here to make mudras your own, to use them as utensils for savoring the preciousness of your own experience. May you enjoy exploring the multi-faceted world of mudras contained between these pages as much as we have enjoyed bringing this book to fruition.

Om Shanti Shanti Shanti

THE
MUDRAS

ABHAYA MUDRA I

अभयमुद्रा

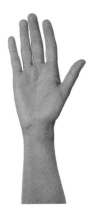

English "fearless" or "fear not"

Devanagari अभयमुद्रा

Transliteration Abhayamudrā

* **Description** *Abhaya Mudra I* is a single-hand gesture (*asamyukta hasta*) common to the yoga tradition. It is referred to as the "seal of fearlessness" and is used in Hinduism, Indian Tantrism, and Buddhism. The mudra is most commonly employed as a gesture of protection and pacification in ritual practice and in iconographic depictions of deities, sages, and saints. It is used to dispel fear and to evoke the direct experience of Openness.[1] It also represents the Five Elements[2] resting in their natural relationship, with the center of the palm as the *bindu*, or central point of focus.

* **Technique** Raise the right hand in front of your right shoulder, palm facing forward, slightly cupped, with the fingers extending upward. Keep your shoulder relaxed, elbow bent, and hand still. Feel the center of your palm warm, as if radiating a soft light. Rest the left hand in your lap with the palm up, or let it hang gently at your side during standing or walking practice.

* **Application** Use *Abhaya Mudra I* during seated meditation and self-reflection when fear and ego clinging arise. Hold the mudra for 5 to 45 minutes. Imagine that whatever causes you fear is looking directly into the center of your upheld palm. Feel that your courage and openness are unwavering, and fear is subdued by the power of your unswerving acceptance. Through regular practice in this way, fear is sublimated into fearlessness.

* **Benefits** Calms the mind, reduces anxiety and inner conflict, removes attachment and aversion to thoughts, emotions, and sensations.

अभयमुद्रा

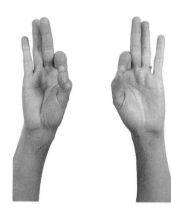

English "fearless" or "fear not"

Devanagari अभयमुद्रा

Transliteration Abhayamudrā

* **Description** *Abhaya Mudra II* is a joint-hand gesture (*samyukta hasta*) used in the yoga tradition. It is common to the *Yoga Tattva Mudra Vijnana* form where it is used to dispel fear and evoke courage.

* **Technique** Join the tips of the thumb and index finger on each hand. Hold the hands palms facing forward at shoulder height.

* **Application** Use *Abhaya Mudra II* during seated meditation or self-reflection when you want to dispel fear and cut through ego clinging. Hold the mudra for 5 to 45 minutes, making sure to keep the shoulders relaxed. Feel that your courage and openness are unwavering. Fear is subdued by the power of your unswerving acceptance.

* **Benefits** Calms the mind, reduces anxiety and inner conflict, removes attachment and aversion to thoughts, emotions, and sensations, bringing one into harmony with the way things naturally are.

Abhaya Hrdaya Mudra
अभयहृदयमुद्रा

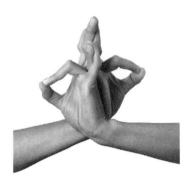

English "fearless heart"

Devanagari अभयहृदयमुद्रा

Transliteration Abhayahṛdayamudrā

❉ **Description** *Abhaya Hrdaya Mudra* is a joint-hand gesture (*samyukta hasta*) used in the yoga tradition as a powerful energy conductor and mind seal. It is a lesser-known Tantric gesture that, according to oral tradition, was traditionally kept secret among initiates. The mudra is known for its unique ability to rejuvenate one's vital force and reduce fragmented thoughts and scattered energy.

❉ **Technique** Raise the hands in front of the chest, palms facing center. Cross the wrists with the backs of the hands touching, right hand closest to your body, palms facing to the sides. Firmly interlock the index, middle, and little fingers, while connecting the tips of the thumb and ring finger on both hands, forming two rings.

❉ **Application** In a seated meditation posture, hold the mudra firmly to your chest and pull down gently rooting it into the base of your sternum. Breathe naturally and hold for 5 to 45 minutes.

❉ **Benefits** Nourishes the heart and lungs, improves digestion, imparts a powerful sense of vitality and calm, can help reduce nightmares and reestablish basic sanity to a troubled mind. Use of this mudra is especially helpful during times of exhaustion, healing from debilitating illness, or regaining strength after surgery. Energetically, it allows heat to descend from the head through the chest down into the belly, thus regulating the healthy function of all the internal organs.

NOTE This mudra may be performed lying down (especially in the case of recuperation after surgery or serious illness), but it is important that the upper body be slightly elevated so that the head and chest are higher than the belly. This takes pressure off the heart and regulates blood pressure.

अधोमुखमुद्रा

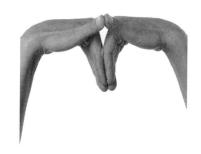

English "downward facing"

Devanagari अधोमुखमुद्रा

Transliteration Adhomukhamudrā

✤ **Description** *Adhomukha Mudra* is a joint-hand gesture (*samyukta hasta*) used in the yoga tradition for healing, especially cancer. It is part of the *Yoga Tattva Mudra Vijnana* form, and is one of the traditional thirty-two *Gayatri Mudras*, specifically the tenth gesture in the sub-set of twenty-four mudras practiced before meditation or recitation of the *Gayatri Mantra*.

✤ **Technique** Join the tips of the thumbs together with the palms facing downward. Point all the other fingers down while resting the tops of the fingers and first knuckles together. Keep all fingers straight and relaxed. Hold the mudra at the level of the waist, thumbs just in front of the navel.

✤ **Application** In a comfortable meditation posture, hold the mudra for 2 to 5 minutes while focusing on the navel and evoking the sense of warmth and rootedness. For healing, especially serious illness such as cancer, hold the mudra for 20 to 45 minutes, two to three sessions per day is ideal.

✤ **Benefits** Activates the digestive fire, increases transformative and self-healing powers, reduces toxicity, readies the mind for meditation, prayer, or recitation of mantas.

NOTE For women practicing during their menstrual cycle, move the position of the mudra to the heart center, with the tips of the thumbs lightly touching the base of the sternum.

ADHOMUSHTI MUKULA MUDRA
अधोमुष्टिमुकुलमुद्रा

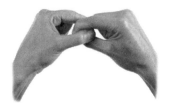

English "downward-fist-closed"

Devanagari अधोमुष्टिमुकुलमुद्रा

Transliteration Adhomuṣṭimukulamudrā

◈ **Description** *Adhomushti Mukula Mudra* is a joint-hand gesture (*samyukta hasta*) common to the dance tradition. In the *Abhinaya Darpana*, it is noted as one of the gestures that indicate "wild animals."

◈ **Technique** With the palms facing each other, fold your little, ring, and middle fingers into the palm. Forming two interlocking rings, connect the tips of the thumb and the index finger of each hand.

◈ **Application** Used in the dance tradition to denote a monkey.

अग्निमुद्रा

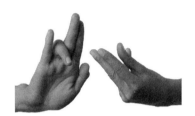

English "god of fire"

Devanagari अग्निमुद्रा

Transliteration Agnimudrā

Additional Name *Vahni*

- **Description** *Agni Mudra* is a joint-hand gesture (*samyukta hasta*) used by performing artists. It is found in the traditional set of sixteen *Deva Hastas*, denoting Hindu gods and goddesses as described in the *Abhinaya Darpana*. It indicates the form and character of the Hindu deity *Agni*.

- **Technique** Assume *Kangula Mudra* (p.104) with your left hand, and *Tripataka Mudra* (p.253) with your right, held at shoulder height.

- **Application** It is used to indicate *Agni*, the Hindu god of fire.

NOTE There are several combinations of mudras used to express the various traits and emblems of *Agni Deva*. The most common form is indicated here.

AJNA CHAKRA MUDRA

आज्ञाचक्रमुद्रा

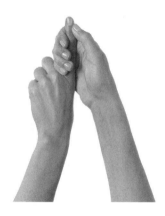

English "command wheel"

Devanagari आज्ञाचक्रमुद्रा

Transliteration Ājñācakramudrā

❋ **Description** *Ajna Chakra Mudra* is a joint-hand gesture (*samyukta hasta*) used in Indian Tantric Yoga and Japanese martial arts to open the "third eye." It employs the relationship of Fire (thumb) and Air (index) Elements to focus attention and intensify energy in an effort to awaken inner vision.

❋ **Technique** Extend the left index finger and curl the other fingers into the palm. Use the left thumb to cover the nails of the other three fingers. Grasp the extended index finger with your right hand, using your right thumb to press gently on the outer corner of the nail bed of the left index finger.

❋ **Application** In a seated meditation posture, hold the mudra in your lap and focus lightly on the space between your eyebrows. For increased intensity, bring the mudra a few inches in front of your forehead, pointing the tip of the extended index finger toward the third eye center. Hold for 1 to 2 minutes, then lower the mudra back into the lap.

❋ **Benefits** Awakens the *Ajna Chakra*, opens spiritual vision, stimulates the pituitary gland, clarifies the mind, improves concentration and intuition.

CAUTION Do not hold the mudra in front of the eyebrow center for more than 2 minutes. This is a powerful mudra that is best learned under the guidance of a competent teacher. If used inappropriately, it can generate excess heat in the head that can be harmful to the brain, eyes, and nervous system.

अलपद्ममुद्रा

English "fully opened lotus"

Devanagari अलपद्ममुद्रा

Transliteration Alapadmamudrā

Additional Names *Sola-padma, Ala-pallava, Chakravaka*

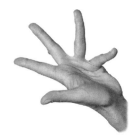

❋ **Description** *Alapadma Mudra* is the twentieth hand gesture of the twenty-eight single-hand mudras (*asamyukta hastas*) as described in the *Abhinaya Darpana*. It is noted in the *Natya Shastra* as *Ala-pallava*. According to mythology, the mudra originates from *Shri Krishna*, referring to the time when he was a young child stealing butter and milk. The associated sage is *Vasanta*, race is *Gandharva*, color is dusky, and deity is *Surya*, the sun.

❋ **Technique** Turn your palm to face upward and stretch all fingers keeping them separated and extended. Turn your little finger toward your palm and fan out the rest of the fingers evenly away from the little finger.

❋ **Application** Primarily used by performing artists to create context and express emotional states or specific actions. *Viniyoga*: *Vikacha-abja* ("a fully bloomed lotus"); *Kapittha-diphala* ("wood apple"); *Avarthaka* ("circular movement"); *Kucha* ("breast"); *Viraha* ("yearning to the beloved"); *Mukura* ("mirror"); *Poorna-chandra* ("full moon"); *Saundarya-bhavana* ("beautiful form"); *Dhamilla* ("hair-knot"); *Chandra-shala* ("moon pavilion"); *Grama* ("village"); *Udru-thakopa* ("great anger"); *Tataka* ("pond" or "lake"); *Shakata* ("cart"); *Chakravaka* ("type of bird"); *Kala-kalarava* ("murmuring sound"); *Slagana* ("praise"). Additional usages are fresh ghee, sweets, head, crown, braided hair, cluster of flowers, ball, dancing, fort, palace, and sweetness.

❋ **Benefits** Stimulates all five fingers and therefore activates all Five Elements in the body, improves circulation and benefits the heart, boosts vitality, and energizes body and mind.

Anahata Chakra Mudra

अनाहतचक्रमुद्रा

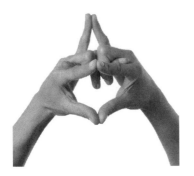

English "wheel of un-struck sound"

Devanagari अनाहतचक्रमुद्रा

Transliteration Anāhatacakramudrā

❋ **Description** *Anahata Mudra* is a complex joint-hand gesture (*samyukta hasta*) used in Tantric Yoga and Japanese martial arts to open the heart center. The mudra beautifully weaves the Five Elements into a *yantra*, a visual symbol representing the essence of potentiality. The Elements of Fire (thumb), Air (index), and Water (little finger) express outwardly, while Ether (middle) and Earth (ring) interlock in the middle of the mudra. *Anahata* means "un-struck sound," and this mudra is a gateway into the silent openness of the human heart.

❋ **Technique** Place the right ring finger in the web of the index/middle of the left hand. Place the left ring finger in the web of the index/middle of the right hand. Curl the middle fingers downward locking the ring fingers into place. Touch the tips of the thumbs, index, and little fingers together and extend them upward.

❋ **Application** In a comfortable seated position, hold the mudra in front of the chest while gazing inwardly at the heart center (at the base of the sternum). Relax the chest, shoulders, and belly. Rest in stillness for 5 to 45 minutes.

❋ **Benefits** Improves the health of the heart, lungs, and breasts, regulates breathing, expands feelings of compassion and love, increases healing abilities.

अङ्गारकमुद्रा

English "planet Mars"

Devanagari अङ्गारकमुद्रा

Transliteration Aṅgarakamudrā

Additional Names *Kuja, Bhauma, Mangala*

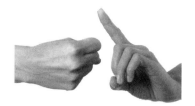

- **Description** *Angaraka Mudra* is a joint-hand gesture (*samyukta hasta*) used by performing artists. It is found in the traditional set of the nine planets (*Nava-Graha Hastas*) as described in the *Abhinaya Darpana*. It indicates the character of the planet Mars.

- **Technique** Assume *Suchi Mudra* (p.240) with your left hand and *Mushti Mudra* (p.163) with your right hand. Place your hands in front of your chest and stand in *sama* position (straight and elongated posture). Evoke a fierce gaze.

- **Application** To denote the planet Mars.

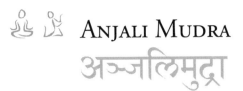

ANJALI MUDRA
अञ्जलिमुद्रा

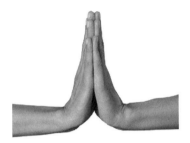

English "prayer" or "salutation"

Devanagari अञ्जलिमुद्रा

Transliteration Añjalimudrā

◈ **Description** *Anjali Mudra* is commonly used in yoga and Indian dance. It is the first hand gesture of the twenty-four joint-hand mudras (*samyukta hastas*) as described in the *Abhinaya Darpana*. It is also noted in the *Natya Shastra*, *Abhinaya Chandrika*, and *Hasta Lakshana Deepika*.[3] The associated patron deity is *Ksetrapala*.[4]

◈ **Technique** Join the hands palm to palm in front of the chest, with the fingers collected and extended upward.

◈ **Application** *Namaskaram* ("to bow or salute"). Used to bow to deities ("*Devata*"), teachers ("*Guru*"), and highly regarded people ("*Vipranam*"). The gesture is held above the head for deities, in front of the face for elders and teachers, and in front of the chest for general respect. It is also used to show obedience, to clap a beat, to indicate the form of *Shiva*, for meditation, and to await instruction from one's guru. *Anjali Mudra* is used extensively as part of the spiritual cultures of East and West as a gesture of prayer, to show respect, humble oneself, and surrender to the greatness of life.

◈ **Benefits** Calming and centering, facilitates connection to the heart and central channel (*sushumna-nadi*), evokes feelings of humility, reverence, and devotion.

अपानमुद्रा

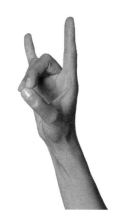

English "downward moving air" or "downward force"

Devanagari अपानमुद्रा

Transliteration Apānamudrā

❋ **Description** *Apana Mudra* is a single-hand gesture (*asamyukta hasta*) common to the *Yoga Tattva Mudra Vijnana* form. It is used in the yogic tradition to regulate the downward rooting energy in the body; the energetic force governing elimination and purification.

❋ **Technique** Join the tips of the ring and middle fingers together with the thumb. Keep the index and little finger extended.

❋ **Application** In a comfortable seated position, form the mudra with each hand and rest the hands on the thighs. Soften the belly and breath naturally. Move your attention to the navel center. Smile inwardly and hold for 5 to 45 minutes.

❋ **Benefits** General detoxifying effect on the body, improves elimination, reduces constipation, benefits the urinary bladder and uterus, regulates menstruation, and clarifies the skin.

NOTE To increase the self-healing effects of this mudra, practice 2 to 3 sessions per day. In the last month of pregnancy the mudra may be used to improve tone and suppleness of the pelvic girdle and birth canal, thereby assisting ease of delivery.

CAUTION *Apana Mudra* is contraindicated in the first eight months of pregnancy.

ARALA MUDRA

अरलमुद्रा

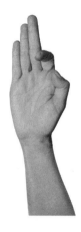

English "bent" or "crooked"

Devanagari अरलमुद्रा

Transliteration Aralamudrā

☸ **Description** *Arala Mudra* is the seventh hand gesture of the twenty-eight single-hand mudras (*asamyukta hastas*) as described in the *Abhinaya Darpana*. It is also noted in the *Natya Shastra* and *Hasta Lakshana Deepika*. According to mythology, this mudra originated from the sage *Agastya*[5] while he was drinking the seven seas. Its color is red, race is mixed, and patron deity is *Vasudeva.*[6]

☸ **Technique** Hold your hand facing outward with all fingers collected and pointing upward, including the thumb. Bend your index finger 90 degrees at the middle joint.

☸ **Application** Primarily used by performing artists to create context and express emotional states and specific actions. *Viniyoga*: *Vishadhyam Amritam Panay* ("drinking poison" or "drinking nectar"); *Prachanda Pavana* ("violent wind"); *Aposana* ("sipping water"). Additional expressions include: benediction, loathing a friend, dressing the hair, wiping sweat from the brow, applying kajal to the eyes, a woman's self-admiration, and the courage and dignity of a man.

अर्चकमुद्रा

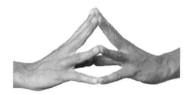

English "worshipping"

Devanagari अर्चकमुद्रा

Transliteration Arcakamudrā

- **Description** *Archaka Mudra* is a joint-hand gesture (*samyukta hasta*) described in the *Abhinaya Chandrika*.[7]

- **Technique** Separate the fingers of each hand and connect the fingertips of the two hands, matching corresponding fingers.

- **Application** Utilized in the dance tradition to express worshipping of deities and expressing respect to divine nature.

- **Benefits** Improves concentration, calms the nerves, balances left and right hemispheres of the brain.

ARDHACHANDRA MUDRA

अर्धचन्द्रमुद्रा

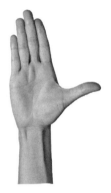

English "half-moon"

Devanagari अर्धचन्द्रमुद्रा

Transliteration Ardhacandramudrā

✦ **Description** *Ardhachandra Mudra* is the sixth hand gesture of the twenty-eight single-hand mudras (*asamyukta hastas*) as described in the *Abhinaya Darpana*. It is also noted in the *Natya Shastra* and the *Abhinaya Chandrika*. According to mythology, this gesture originated from *Shiva's* desire for ornaments, of which the moon is one. The associated sage is *Atri*, race is *Vaishya*, color is smoky, and patron deity is *Mahadeva*.

✦ **Technique** Raise your hand with the palm facing forward, fingers extended upward. Stretch your thumb away from your palm at a 90-degree angle to your fingers. Maintain active fingers and a flat palm.

✦ **Application** Primarily used by performing artists to create context and express emotional states or specific actions. *Viniyoga*: *Krishna-ashtamibhaji-chandray* ("the moon on the eighth day of its waning cycle"); *Gala-hastarthake* ("seizing one by the throat"); *Bhala-yudha* ("spear"); *Devathanam-abishechana-karmani* ("offerings to god"); *Bukpathra* ("eating plate"); *Udbava* ("origin" or "birth"); *Katyam* ("waist"); *Chintayam* ("thinking" or "worrying"); *Athma-vachakam* ("contemplation"); *Dhyana* ("meditation"); *Prathana* ("prayers"); *Anganam-sparsha* ("touching the limbs"); *Prakrutanam-namaskaram* ("greeting common people"). Additional usages of this mudra denote: a bangle, wrist, mirror, astonishment, effort, intemperance, entirety, counting rhythm, tying up the hair, supporting the cheek in grief, elephant ear, expelling evil, wiping sweat from the brow, adolescence, ability, consecration, eyebrow, cloth, bow, preeminence, tightening the girdle, making a vessel, body, movement of the feet, carrying a child, back of the body.

ARDHAMUKULA MUDRA

अर्धमुकुलमुद्रा

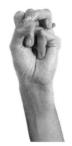

English "half-closed"

Devanagari अर्धमुकुलमुद्रा

Transliteration Ardhamukulamudrā

- **Description** *Ardhamukula Mudra* is a single-hand gesture (*asamyukta hasta*) common to the dance tradition. In the *Abhinaya Darpana*, it is noted as one of the gestures that indicate "wild animals."

- **Technique** Fold the little, middle, and index fingers into the palm. Join the tips of the ring finger and thumb.

- **Application** Used in the dance tradition to denote a cat.

ARDHAPATAKA MUDRA
अर्धपताकमुद्रा

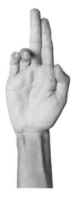

English "half-flag"

Devanagari अर्धपताकमुद्रा

Transliteration Ardhapatākamudrā

❀ **Description** *Ardhapataka Mudra* is the third hand gesture of the twenty-eight single-hand mudras (*asamyukta hastas*) as described in the *Abhinaya Darpana*. It is also found in Buddhist and Hindu ritual and art depicting or evoking a deity.

❀ **Technique** Raise your hand to face outward with your fingers collected and extended upward. Bend your thumb slightly to touch the base of the index finger. Bend the ring and little finger 90 degrees at the middle joint.

❀ **Application** Primarily used by performing artists to create context and express emotional states and specific actions. *Viniyoga*: *Pallava* ("tender leaf" or "new growth"); *Phalaka* ("wooden plank" or "panel for drawing"); *Theera* ("river bank"); *Ubayoo-rithi-Vachaka* ("two" or "two people together"); *Krakacha* ("saw"); *Churi-kayancha* ("pocket knife"); *Dvaja* ("temple flag"); *Gopura-sringayoh* ("horns on top of temple tower).

ARDHARECHITA MUDRA

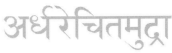

अर्धरेचितमुद्रा

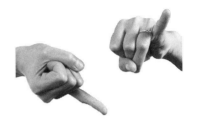

English "half-contraction of the eyebrow"

Devanagari अर्धरेचितमुद्रा

Transliteration Ardharecitamudrā

※ **Description** *Ardharechita Mudra* is a joint-hand gesture (*samyukta hasta*) common to the dance tradition. It is noted in the *Abhinaya Darpana*. The patron deity associated with it is *Nandikeshvara*.

※ **Technique** With each hand, fold the index, middle, and ring fingers under the thumb, while stretching the little finger upward. Turn your right palm to face upward, left downward. Keep your hands in front of your torso about 6 inches from the body.

※ **Application** Used by performing artists to denote invitation, giving gifts, and concealing actions.

ARDHASUCHI MUDRA
अर्धसुचिमुद्रा

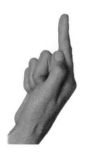

English "sprout"

Devanagari अर्धसुचिमुद्रा

Transliteration Ardhasucimudrā

Additional Names *Ardhasuchika, Tambula*

* **Description** *Ardhasuchi Mudra* is a single-hand gesture (*asamyukta hasta*) noted in the *Abhinaya Chandrika*.

* **Technique** Extend your index finger upward, touching the tip of the thumb to the middle joint of the index finger. The middle, ring, and little fingers are folded into the palm.

* **Application** Used by performing artists to denote a sprout, young bird, or large insect.

ASHVARATNA MUDRA

अश्वरत्नमुद्रा

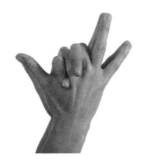

English "horse-jewel"

Devanagari अश्वरत्नमुद्रा

Transliteration Aśvaratnamudrā

* **Description** *Ashvaratna Mudra* is a joint-hand gesture (*samyukta hasta*) common to the *Vajrayana* Buddhist tradition where it is employed in ritual associated with the goddess *Tara*. It also denotes the "Precious Horse," one of the Seven Jewels of Royal Power (*Saptaratna*).[8]

* **Technique** Join the palms together with the index and rings fingers interlaced. Extend the thumbs, ring fingers, and little fingers. Maintain space in the web between the ring and little fingers.

* **Application** In a comfortable seated position, hold the mudra in front of the chest. Relax your shoulders and breathe naturally. Imagine you are mounting a mythical horse that gallops high into the sky, giving you a clear view of your entire life. With this "bird's eye view," notice what behaviors in your life are not serving your highest potential. Gathering your determination, renounce any negative habits once and for all, recommitting yourself to a life of spiritual cultivation with new resolve. Hold for 5 to 45 minutes.

* **Benefits** Balances Earth, Water, and Fire Elements, benefiting digestion, circulation, and overall vitality. Cuts through ego clinging and narrow-mindedness, gives new perspective on your choices and life's path.

Avahana Mudra

अवहनमुद्रा

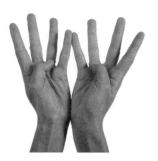

English "invitation" or "invocation"

Devanagari अवहनमुद्रा

Transliteration Avahanamudrā

Additional Name *Avahani*

❋ **Description** *Avahana Mudra* is a joint-hand gesture (*samyukta hasta*) common to the Hindu tradition where it is used as a ritual gesture to summon the presence of a deity.

❋ **Technique** Raise the hand in front of the face, palms facing you, with the sides of the hands touching. Place the tips of the thumbs to the base of the ring fingers. Keep the outer tips of the little finger pads touching, as you splay all of the fingers.

❋ **Application** In a comfortable seated position, hold the mudra about a foot from your face. Relax the shoulders and chest, and breathe naturally. Concentrating on your chosen form of divinity (*ishta devata*) or a specific divine quality, mentally invite this presence into your heart. Generate feelings of devotion, altruism, and sincerity. Hold for 5 to 45 minutes.

❋ **Benefits** Grounding and centering, improves digestion and assimilation, strengthens devotion and connection with one's personal deity or principle of divinity, truth, etc.

NOTE Using *Avahana Mudra* in conjunction with a mantra related to the deity or object of concentration you have selected can greatly enhance the effects of the practice. For general use, the seed mantra Om may be used.

अवहितमुद्रा

English "dissimulation" or "holding things"

Devanagari अवहितमुद्रा

Transliteration Avahitamudrā

Additional names *Lalita, Udveshtitalapadma*

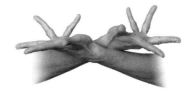

❉ **Description** *Avahita Mudra* is the twenty-fourth hand gesture of the twenty-four joint-hand mudras (*samyukta hastas*) as described in the *Abhinaya Darpana*. It is noted in the *Natya Shastra* as a different variation (see "technique" below). Its patron deity is *Markandeya*.[9]

❉ **Technique** Cross two *Alapadma Mudras* (p.41) in front of your chest. The variation noted in the *Natya Shastra* employs crossed *Shukatunda Mudras* (p.228) with the fingers turned to point downward.

❉ **Application** Primarily used by performing artists to create context and express emotional states or specific actions. *Viniyoga*: *Sringara-natana* ("erotic dance"); *Lilakanduka-dharana* ("holding a ball while playing"); *Kucha-artha* ("breasts"). The *Shukatunda* variation from *Natya Shastra* denotes weakness, sigh, revealing one's body, thinness, and yearning for the beloved.

Note The word *lalita* means "graceful elegance." The *Lalita Mudra* version is held above the head and its patron deity is *Vaishnavi*. It denotes a *sala* tree, fort, and mountain.

BADHA MUDRA

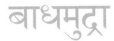

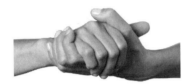

English "suffering"

Devanagari बाधमुद्रा

Transliteration Bādhamudrā

❋ **Description** *Badha Mudra* is a joint-hand gesture (*samyukta hasta*) noted in the *Abhinaya Chandrika*.

❋ **Technique** Clasp the hands together with the fingers firmly cupped.

❋ **Application** Utilized in the dance tradition to express suffering or disturbance, as well as pleading for help in the form of divine intervention.

बकमुद्रा

English "crane"

Devanagari बकमुद्रा

Transliteration Bakamudrā

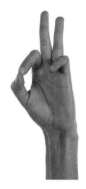

✦ **Description** *Baka Mudra* is a single-hand gesture (*asamyukta hasta*) common to the dance tradition. In the *Abhinaya Darpana*, it is noted as one of the gestures used to indicate "flying creatures." Also known as the "mingled *Hamsa* (swan)."

✦ **Technique** Join the tips of the index finger and thumb. Extend the middle and ring fingers upward, and fold the little finger down toward the palm.

✦ **Application** Used in the dance tradition to denote a crane and other birds.

Bam Mudra

बंमुद्रा

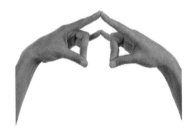

English "to bind"

Devanagari बंमुद्रा

Transliteration Baṁmudrā

* **Description** *Bam Mudra* is a lesser-known joint-hand gesture (*samyukta hasta*) used in Tantric Buddhism (*Vajrayana*) during ritual invocation of the goddess *Tara*. The mudra gets its name from the third syllable of the related mantra "*Jah Hum Bam Hoh*," usually preceded by "*Om A Hum*," and chanted in conjunction with the use of the mudra as a ritual offering.

* **Technique** Join the tips of the middle and ring fingers together with the pad of the thumb (both hands are identical). Lightly touch the tips of the index and little fingers, and hold the mudra in front of the throat.

* **Application** In a comfortable seated position, hold the mudra for 5 to 45 minutes with the shoulders relaxed. Relax and release all interest in gaining results, remaining open to the inherent wisdom expressing spontaneously.

* **Benefits** Evokes the qualities of openness and acceptance. Used in conjunction with regular meditation practice, this mudra can reveal how the virtuous qualities of the various deities, in this case namely *Tara*, are inherent in our own original nature.

CAUTION The mudras and mantras used in *Vajrayana* are best learned under the guidance of a qualified teacher.

बाणमुद्रा

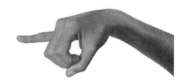

English "arrow"

Devanagari बाणमुद्रा

Transliteration Bāṇamudrā

Additional names *Teera*

※ **Description** *Bana Mudra* is a single-hand gesture (*asamyukta hasta*) noted in the *Abhinaya Chandrika*.

※ **Technique** Extend the little finger upward and cover the nails of the ring, middle, and index fingers with the thumb.

※ **Application** Used to denote the number six, beautiful eye, and an arrow.

BHAIRAVA MUDRA

भैरवमुद्रा

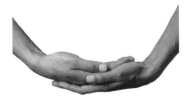

English "fierce," "terrifying," or "beyond fear of death"

Devanagari भैरवमुद्रा

Transliteration Bhairavamudrā

❋ **Description** *Bhairava Mudra* is a joint-hand gesture (*samyukta hasta*) common to the yoga tradition. It represents the force responsible for the dissolution of the universe, personified as Lord *Shiva*. The left and right hands represent the *ida* and *pingala nadis* respectively, the lunar and solar energy channels within the body. Joined together, the hands symbolize the innate union of the individual and supreme consciousness.

❋ **Technique** Place the right hand on top of the left, and rest both hands in the lap, palms up. Keep all fingers lightly collected, including the thumbs.

❋ **Application** In a comfortable seated position, rest the mudra in your lap. If seated in a chair, a cloth may be placed over your lap to provide a stable surface for the mudra to rest upon. Lengthen the spine, soften the belly and chest, and lightly close the eyes. In relaxed stillness, hold the mudra for 5 to 45 minutes.

❋ **Benefits** Calms the mind, serves as an aid to meditation, cuts ego clinging, and imparts the courage needed to fully embrace life as it is.

NOTE The female counterpart to *Bhairava Mudra* is called *Bhairavi Mudra*, and is formed by placing the left palm on top of the right. Other details of the practice are the same. *Bhairavi Mudra* expresses the fierce aspect of the goddess and also symbolizes a female adept of Tantric Yoga.

BHARTRI MUDRA

भर्तृमुद्रा

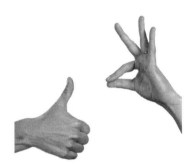

English "husband"

Devanagari भर्तृमुद्रा

Transliteration Bhartṛmudrā

   ❋ **Description** *Bhartri Mudra* is a joint-hand gesture (*samyukta hasta*) used by performing artists. It is found in the traditional set of the eleven relationships (*Bandava Hastas*) as described in the *Abhinaya Darpana*. It indicates husband.

   ❋ **Technique** Assume *Hamsasya Mudra* (p.96) with your left hand and *Shikhara Mudra* (p.225) with your right hand, held by the throat.

   ❋ **Application** This gesture denotes husband.

Bhartri Bhratri Mudra

भर्तृभ्रातृमुद्रा

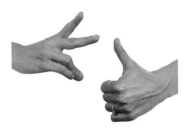

English "brother-in-law"

Devanagari भर्तृभ्रातृमुद्रा

Transliteration Bhartṛbhrātṛmudrā

※ **Description** *Bhartri Bhratri Mudra* is a joint-hand gesture (*samyukta hasta*) used by performing artists. It is found in the traditional set of the eleven relationships (*Bandava Hastas*) as described in the *Abhinaya Darpana*. It indicates brother-in-law.

※ **Technique** Assume *Shikhara Mudra* (p.225) with your left hand and *Kartarimukha Mudra I* (p.115) with your right hand. Hold your hands in front of your body or by your side.

※ **Application** To denote a brother-in-law.

BHERUNDA MUDRA

भेरुण्डमुद्रा

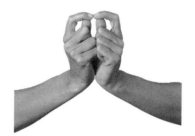

English "pair of birds" or "two-headed bird"

Devanagari भेरुण्डमुद्रा

Transliteration Bheruṇḍamudrā

❋ **Description** *Bherunda Mudra* is the twenty-third hand gesture of the twenty-four joint-hand mudras (*samyukta hastas*) as described in the *Abhinaya Darpana*.

❋ **Technique** Form *Kapittha Mudra* (p.106) with each hand, joining the inner wrists in front of your chest. A variation of this mudra is performed with the wrists across from each other, so the *Kapittha* hands are back to back.

❋ **Application** Used to denote the *Bherunda*, which is a two-headed mythological bird of Hindu mythology. *Bherunda* is considered a fierce creature, and is the form that *Narasimha* (the half-lion incarnation of *Vishnu*) turned into during his epic battle with the demon.

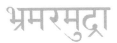 # Bhramara Mudra

भ्रमरमुद्रा

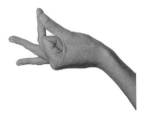

English "bee"

Devanagari भ्रमरमुद्रा

Transliteration Bhramaramudrā

* **Description** *Bhramara Mudra* is used in yoga and in Classical Indian Dance. It is the twenty-second hand gesture of the twenty-eight single-hand mudras (*asamyukta hastas*) as described in the *Abhinaya Darpana*. It is also noted in the *Natya Shastra*. According to mythology, it originated from *Kashyapa*, while he was preparing earrings for his wife *Aditi*.[10] The associated sage is *Kapila*, race is *Khachara*, color is black, and patron deity is *Garuda*.

* **Technique** Curl your index finger toward the base of the thumb. Touch the tip of the thumb to the first crease of the middle finger. The ring and little fingers remain extended.

* **Application (yoga)** In a comfortable seated position, form the mudra with both hands, resting the hands in your lap, palms up. Soften the chest and diaphragm, feel the ribs move freely as you breathe in a natural rhythm (do not try to control the breath). In relaxed stillness, hold it for 5 to 45 minutes. To increase the healing potential, or in the case of acute symptoms, practice it 3 to 5 sessions per day.

* **Application (dance)** Primarily used by performing artists to create context and express emotional states or specific actions. *Viniyoga*: *Bhramara* ("bee"); *Shuka* ("parrot"); *Yoga* ("union"); *Paksha* ("wing of a bird"); *Sarasa* ("crane"); *Kokila* ("cuckoo"). Additional usages denote: vow of silence, horn, elephant tusk, picking flowers, whispering a secret, removing a thorn, and untying a belt.

* **Benefits** Improves the health of the lungs and large intestine, balances the immune system (particularly in cases of immune over-reaction), reduces allergic reactions to food and pollen, soothes cough and irritated lungs.

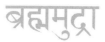

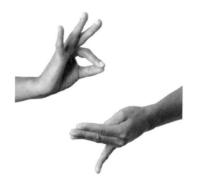

English "supreme or absolute god of creation"

Devanagari ब्रह्ममुद्रा

Transliteration Brahmamudrā

❋ **Description** *Brahma Mudra* is a joint-hand gesture (*samyukta hasta*) used by performing artists. It is found in the traditional set of sixteen *Deva Hastas*, denoting Hindu gods and goddesses as described in the *Abhinaya Darpana*. It indicates the form and character of the Hindu deity *Brahma*.

❋ **Technique** Assume *Chatura Mudra* (p.73) with your left hand and *Hamsasya Mudra* (p.96) with your right. The *Chatura* hand is turned palm upward and held in front of the waist, while the *Hamsasya* hand is held in front of the heart center.

❋ **Application** Used to indicate *Brahma*, the Hindu god of creation. Stand with your feet apart and keep your hand gestures about 6 inches away from your body. The hand formation indicates writing with the right hand onto a book held by the left hand. This symbolizes the power of creation.

NOTE *There are several combinations of mudras used to express the various traits and emblems of Brahma Deva. The one indicated here appears to be the most common.*

Budha Mudra

बुधमुद्रा

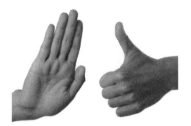

English "planet Mercury"

Devanagari बुधमुद्रा

Transliteration Budhamudrā

Additional Name *Soumya*

❋ **Description** *Budha Mudra* is a joint-hand gesture (*samyukta hasta*) used by performing artists. It is found in the traditional set of the nine planets (*Nava-Graha Hastas*) as described in the *Abhinaya Darpana*. It indicates the character of the planet Mercury.

❋ **Technique** Assume *Mushti* (p.163) or *Shikhara Mudra* (p.225) with your left hand and *Pataka Mudra* (p.186) with your right hand. Place your hands in front of your chest and stand in *sama* position (straight and elongated posture). Assume a satisfied and pleasant gaze.

❋ **Application** To denote the planet Mercury.

CANCUKA MUDRA

चञ्चुकमुद्रा

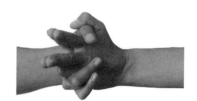

English "bird's beak"

Devanagari चञ्चुकमुद्रा

Transliteration Cañcukamudrā

❀ **Description** *Cancuka Mudra* is a joint-hand gesture (*samyukta hasta*) common to the dance tradition.

❀ **Technique** Place your hands palm to palm in front of your face. Cross your thumbs, ring, and little fingers. Keep your middle and index fingers extended and pressed together. The tips of the index and middle fingers point outward and separate to resemble a bird's beak.

❀ **Application** Used in the dance tradition to express the beak of *Garuda*, an eagle, or other birds.

CHAKRA MUDRA I

चक्रमुद्रा

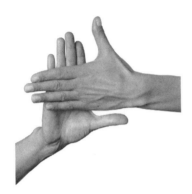

English "wheel" or "discus"

Devanagari चक्रमुद्रा

Transliteration Cakramudrā

❋ **Description** *Chakra Mudra I* is the thirteenth hand gesture of the twenty-four joint-hand mudras (*samyukta hastas*) as described in the *Abhinaya Darpana*.

❋ **Technique** Both hands form *Ardhachandra Mudra* (p.48). Hold the right hand with the palm facing outward, fingers pointing upward at your right side. Place the left hand across the right, palm facing you.

❋ **Application** Primarily used by performing artists to create context and express emotional states or specific actions. *Viniyoga*: *Chakra* ("discus" or "wheel"), which symbolizes *Vishnu*. The *chakra*, a sharp, spinning discus-like weapon, known as *Sudarshana*, is held in *Vishnu's* upper right hand, symbolizing a purified mind.

NOTE The name *Sudarshana* is derived from two words—*Su*, which means good, superior, and *Darshana*, which means vision or sight. Together this implies "superior vision," or seeing the true nature of reality. This mudra represents destruction of one's ignorance and realization of one's true nature.

चक्रमुद्रा

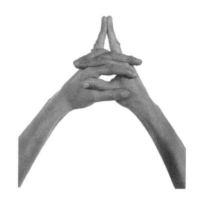

English "wheel"

Devanagari चक्रमुद्रा

Transliteration Cakramudrā

- **Description** *Chakra Mudra II* is a joint-hand gesture (*samyukta hasta*) ritual mudra used in the Indian Tantric tradition and in Japanese Buddhism (*Vajrayana* tradition), where it is employed by priests as a gesture of offering.

- **Technique** Interlace the fingers of both hands. Extend the ring fingers, touching the tips of the two fingers together.

- **Application** In a comfortable seated position, hold the mudra in front of the navel. Soften the belly and breathe naturally. Feel the belly grow warm, as if the sun is shining inside your abdomen. Hold for 5 to 45 minutes.

- **Benefits** Centering and grounding, improves digestion, assimilation and elimination, reduces gas and bloating, increases vigor and self-confidence.

CHAKRAVAKA MUDRA

चक्रवाकमुद्रा

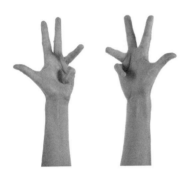

English "a type of bird"

Devanagari चक्रवाकमुद्रा

Transliteration Cakravākamudrā

❋ **Description** *Chakravaka Mudra* is a joint-hand gesture (*samyukta hasta*) common to the dance tradition. In the *Abhinaya Darpana*, it is noted as one of the gestures that indicate "birds."

❋ **Technique** With the palms facing outward, form *Alapadma Mudra* (p.41) with each hand. Hold your hands about 6 inches in front of your body.

❋ **Application** Used by performing artists to denote birds.

Chandra Mudra

चन्द्रमुद्रा

English "Moon"

Devanagari चन्द्रमुद्रा

Transliteration Candramudrā

Additional names *Nisakara, Rajanikara, Sudhakara, Indu, Soma*

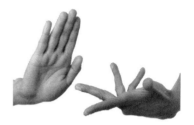

❅ **Description** *Chandra Mudra* is a joint-hand gesture (*samyukta hasta*) used by performing artists. It is found in the traditional set of the nine planets (*Nava-Graha Hastas*) as described in the *Abhinaya Darpana*. It indicates the character of the Moon.

❅ **Technique** Assume *Alapadma Mudra* (p.41) with your left hand and *Pataka Mudra* (p.186) with your right hand. Place your hands by your shoulders and stand in *sama* position (straight and elongated posture). Keep your gaze natural and directed upward.

❅ **Application** To denote the Moon.

NOTE In addition to the basic moon gesture above, there are different formations to denote the rising moon (*bala chandra*) and the full moon (*purna chandra*) as noted in the *Abhinaya Darpana*.[11]

CHANDRAKALA MUDRA

चन्द्रकलामुद्रा

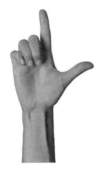

English "crescent moon"

Devanagari चन्द्रकलामुद्रा

Transliteration Candrakalāmudrā

- **Description** *Chandrakala Mudra* is the fourteenth hand gesture of the twenty-eight single-hand mudras (*asamyukta hastas*) as described in the *Abhinaya Darpana*.

- **Technique** Bend the little, ring, and middle fingers into the palm. Extend the index finger and thumb, forming a 90-degree angle.

- **Application** Primarily used in dance and theater to create context and express emotional states or specific actions. *Viniyoga*: *Chandra* ("Moon"); *Mukha* ("face"); *Pradesha* ("the distance between the tip of the index finger and the thumb"); *Shivasya Makuta* ("*Shiva's* crown"); *Ganganadyam* ("river Ganges"); *Laguda* ("axe" or "cane").

- **Benefits** Stimulates the lungs, opens the airways, tones the large intestine, relieves constipation.

CHATURA MUDRA

चतुरमुद्रा

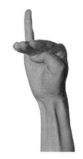

English "jackal" or "clever"

Devanagari चतुरमुद्रा

Transliteration Caturamudrā

⬦ **Description** *Chatura Mudra* is the twenty-first hand gesture of the twenty-eight single-hand mudras (*asamyukta hastas*) as described in the *Abhinaya Darpana*. It is also noted in the *Natya Shastra*. According to mythology, when *Garuda* wished to acquire the nectar of immortality, he sought the permission of his father, *Kashyapa*. *Kashyapa* held *Chatura Mudra* as a sign of granting him permission. The associated sage is *Valakhilya*, race is mixed, color is variegated, and patron deity is *Garuda*. In the Hindu tradition this gesture is also known as *Chaturahasta*, and Shiva holds it in his form *Chaturatandava*.[12]

⬦ **Technique** Hold your hand with the palm facing downward, little finger extended upward, index, middle, and ring fingers held at 90 degrees to the little finger. The thumb is bent under the fingers to touch the base of the ring finger (on the palm side).

⬦ **Application** In the Hindu tradition, it is used to denote a crafty enemy or a panderer. *Shiva Nataraj* is depicted holding this mudra to dispel danger and provide protection. In the dance and theater tradition, it is used to denote the following *Viniyoga*: *Kasturi* ("musk"); *Kimchidartha Swarna-tamra-adi-lohaka* ("some gold, copper, iron, etc."); *Ardra* ("wetness"); *Bhede* ("sorrow"); *Rasa-svada* ("aesthetic pleasure"); *Lochana* ("eyes"); *Varna-bhedana* ("difference in caste or color"); *Sarasa* ("playful converse"); *Pramana* ("oath"); *Mandagamana* ("slow stroll"); *Shakalikrita* ("shuttering" or "piercing"); *Asana* ("seat"); *Ghrita-taila-adau* ("ghee, oil, etc."). Additional usages denote: dust, concentration, camphor, earring, face, forehead, side glance, beloved, cleverness, mirror, precious stones, sufficient, moderate quantity, sword, and cheek.

CHATURASRA MUDRA I

चतुरस्रमुद्रा

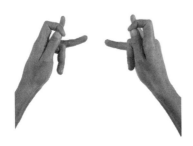

English "square"

Devanagari चतुरस्रमुद्रा

Transliteration Caturasramudrā

❁ **Description** *Chaturasra Mudra I* is a joint-hand gesture (*samyukta hasta*) common to the dance tradition. It is noted in the *Abhinaya Darpana*. The patron deity associated with it is *Varahi*.[13]

❁ **Technique** Form *Katakamukha Mudra III* (p.122) with both hands and hold them directly in front of your chest with the shoulders and elbows relaxed, hands facing each other.

❁ **Application** This gesture is used in dance and theatre to denote the following: churning, holding, milking, covering with cloth, wearing a necklace, dragging rope, tying the girdle or bodice, holding flowers, using a fly-whisk.

CHATURASRA MUDRA II

चतुरस्रमुद्रा

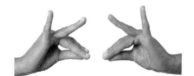

English "square"

Devanagari चतुरस्रमुद्रा

Transliteration Caturasramudrā

⁕ **Description** *Chaturasra Mudra II* is a joint-hand gesture (*samyukta hasta*) common to the dance tradition. It is noted in the *Natya Shastra*.

⁕ **Technique** Form *Katakamukha Mudra I* (p.120) with both hands and hold them directly in front of your chest with the shoulders and elbows relaxed, hands facing each other.

⁕ **Application** See *Chaturasra Mudra I*.

CHATURMUKHA MUDRA
चतुर्मुखमुद्रा

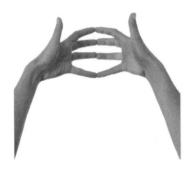

English "four faces" or "four-faced"

Devanagari चतुर्मुखमुद्रा

Transliteration Caturmukhamudrā

❋ **Description** *Chaturmukha Mudra* is a joint-hand gesture (*samyukta hasta*) common to the yoga tradition. It is found in the *Yoga Tattva Mudra Vijnana* form, and is one of the traditional thirty-two *Gayatri Mudras*, specifically the seventh gesture in the sub-set of twenty-four mudras practiced before meditation or recitation of the *Gayatri Mantra*.

❋ **Technique** Lightly touch the tips of the index, middle, ring, and little fingers. The thumbs remain apart.

❋ **Application** In a comfortable seated position, hold the mudra in front of the solar plexus. Relax the chest and shoulders, and breathe naturally. Hold for 5 to 45 minutes.

❋ **Benefits** Readies the mind for meditation, increases feelings of devotion, generosity and surrender, harmonizes Air, Ether, Earth, and Water Elements, while calming the spirit and tempering the heart.

NOTE Many mudras, *Chaturmukha Mudra* included, are traditionally used in flow sequences involving numerous hand positions done in procession. Used as part of a set, the power and effect of mudras can be increased. See Appendix B.

चिन्मुद्रा

English "gesture of consciousness"

Devanagari चिन्मुद्रा

Transliteration Cinmudrā

Additional Name *Vitarka* (name used in Buddhist iconography)

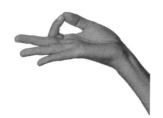

❋ **Description** *Chin Mudra* is perhaps the most commonly used single-hand gesture (*asamyukta hasta*) in the yoga tradition. Its name comes from the Sanskrit word *chit*, meaning "consciousness." The middle, ring, and little fingers symbolize the three *gunas*: *rajas* "activity," *tamas* "inertia," and *sattva* "luminosity." The index finger represents individual consciousness, the thumb universal consciousness. Their joining together in *Chin Mudra* expresses the union, or yoga, of these two aspects. This union is considered the crowning jewel of yoga practice.

❋ **Technique** Lightly join the tip of the index finger with the tip of the thumb. Keep the remaining fingers extended and relaxed.

❋ **Application** In a comfortable seated position, form the mudra with both hands and rest the hands on the thighs, palms up. Relax the chest and shoulders, and breathe naturally. Hold for 5 to 45 minutes.

❋ **Benefits** Evokes the feeling of lightness, calms the mind and brightens the spirit, opens the chest and facilitates diaphragmatic breathing, reverses the outward flow of *prana* and directs energy back toward the body, increases the benefits of any *asana* (yogic position).

NOTE *Chin Mudra* and *Jnana Mudra* look identical and are used interchangeably in many schools of yoga. The distinction occurs when the mudra is placed on the thighs or knees during seated meditation practice: palms up, the gesture is referred to as *Chin Mudra*; palms down, it is known as *Jnana Mudra*. The former produces subtle feelings of lightness, the latter a sense of rootedness.

CHONMUKHA MUKHA MUDRA
चोन्मुखमुखमुद्रा

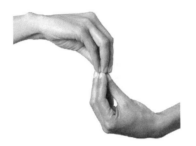

English "up and down face" or "face up and face down"

Devanagari चोन्मुखमुखमुद्रा

Transliteration Conmukhamukhamudrā

Additional Name *Unmukhonmukham*

Description *Chonmukha Mukha Mudra* is a joint-hand gesture (*samyukta hasta*) common to the yoga tradition. It is found in the *Yoga Tattva Mudra Vijnana* form, and is one of the traditional thirty-two *Gayatri Mudras*, specifically the fifteenth gesture in the sub-set of twenty-four mudras practiced before meditation or recitation of the *Gayatri Mantra*.

Technique Collect the fingers of each hand so that the pads of the thumbs lightly touch the pads of the other four fingers. With the left hand facing down, right hand facing up, touch the two mudras together at the fingertips. Hold. Then rotate the hands so that the right hand faces down and the left hand faces up. Hold.

Application In a comfortable seated position, hold the mudra a few inches in front of the chest or solar plexus. Relax the shoulders and breathe naturally. Begin with the left hand facing down and the right facing up. Hold for 5 to 10 minutes. Keeping the tips of the fingers collected, and the two hands touching, rotate the mudras, bringing the right hand on top and left hand below. Hold for 5 to 10 minutes.

Benefits Calms the mind, ignites feelings of devotion, balances solar and lunar energies in the body, harmonizes *apana* and *prana vayus*; is used in yoga therapy to aid cancer treatment and healing of autoimmune diseases.

NOTE Connecting the tip of the tongue with the upper palate during practice of this mudra will significantly increase the benefits. This facilitates a natural balance between rising and descending energies in the body.

दम्पतिमुद्रा

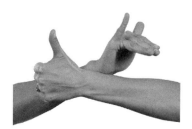

English "husband and wife"

Devanagari दम्पतिमुद्रा

Transliteration Dampatimudrā

* **Description** *Dampati Mudra* is a joint-hand gesture (*samyukta hasta*) used by performing artists. It is found in the traditional set of the eleven relationships (*Bandava Hastas*) as described in the *Abhinaya Darpana*. It indicates husband and wife.

* **Technique** Assume *Shikhara Mudra* (p.225) with your left hand and *Mrigashirsha Mudra* (p.158) with your right hand. Cross the wrists with the left hand held in front. The left and right hand represent male and female respectively.

* **Application** This gesture denotes the union of husband and wife (or, esoterically, the relating of male and female energies).

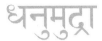

Dhanu Mudra

धनुमुद्रा

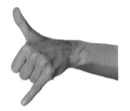

English "bow"

Devanagari धनुमुद्रा

Transliteration Dhanumudrā

❋ **Description** *Dhanu Mudra* is a single-hand gesture (*asamyukta hasta*) noted in the *Abhinaya Chandrika*.

❋ **Technique** Bend the index, middle, and ring fingers into the palm. Stretch the thumb and little fingers away from each other, with the thumb pointing upward and the little finger downward. Hold the hand at arm's length in front of you, resembling holding a bow.

❋ **Application** Typically used in the dance tradition to depict characters holding the bow and arrow such as *Rama*, when he fights *Ravana* to save his wife *Sita*; or *Kamadeva*, the god of love, when he shoots the five flower arrows of the senses; *Shiva* as a hunter; and the goddess as huntress. The bow represents female energy while the arrow (*Bana*) represents the male energy. The bow and arrow represents the power of love and will.

DHARMACHAKRA MUDRA

धर्मचक्रमुद्रा

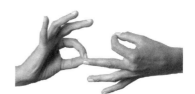

English "wheel of dharma"

Devanagari धर्मचक्रमुद्रा

Transliteration Dharmacakramudrā

❋ **Description** *Dharmachakra Mudra* is a joint-hand gesture (*samyukta hasta*) common to the yoga tradition where it is used to express the insight of alternation, the law of change. Birth and death, night and day, gain and loss, growth and decay, enjoyment and suffering: each of these begets the other in an ongoing cycle. In the Buddhist tradition, the mudra is used to symbolize the "turning of the wheel," or the spreading of the Buddha's teachings (*Buddha Dharma*). Through the practice of contemplation, meditation, and mudras, we can enter a more open and accepting relationship with the law of change. In the words of the *Ashtavakragita*,[14] "Awaken to your own nature, and all delusion melts like a dream." This is the spirit of the *Dharmachakra Mudra*.

❋ **Technique** Join the tips of the thumbs and index fingers of each hand. With the hands in front of your heart, touch the tip of the left middle finger to the tips of the right thumb and index. Your right palm faces forward and your left palm faces your body.

❋ **Application** In a comfortable seated position, hold the mudra in front of your heart center. Breathe naturally and relax your neck, shoulders, and chest. Notice the rhythm of your breathing: the alternation of the in-breath and out-breath. Hold for 5 to 45 minutes.

❋ **Benefits** Opens the chest, facilitates deep breathing, benefits the heart and lungs, balances "inner" and "outer" aspects of life (spiritual and worldly), serves as a window through which we can directly touch the inherent unity behind the veil of duality.

DHVAJA MUSHTI MUDRA

ध्वजमुष्टिमुद्रा

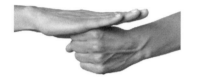

English "flag-fist"

Devanagari ध्वजमुष्टिमुद्रा

Transliteration Dhvajamuṣṭimudrā

* **Description** *Dhvaja Mushti Mudra* is a joint-hand mudra (*samyukta hasta*) noted in the *Abhinaya Chandrika*.

* **Technique** Form a fist with your left hand—bend your fingers inward and place your thumb over the fingers. Place your right palm on top of the fist, palm slightly cupped and facing downward.

* **Application** Used to express keeping a secret, containing a precious item, concealing something, sealing.

ध्यानमुद्रा

English "meditation," "contemplation," or "absorption"

Devanagari ध्यानमुद्रा

Transliteration Dhyānamudrā

Additional names *Samadhi, Dhyanahasta*

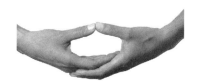

* **Description** *Dhyana Mudra* is a joint-hand gesture (*samyukta hasta*) common to many contemplative traditions throughout Asia. It represents the natural relationship between emptiness and form, and is considered one of the purest expressions of our Original Nature.

* **Technique** Place the left hand in the lap, palm up. Rest the back of the right hand into the palm of the left. Lightly touch the tips of the thumbs together in the shape of a hollow sphere.

* **Application** In a comfortable seated position, place the mudra lightly in the lap. Keep the pressure between the thumbs very gentle, as if holding a piece of paper. Maintain the hollow feeling of the mudra. Relax the shoulders and let the elbows find their natural position. Do not force the elbows forward, as this will cause unnecessary tension in the neck and shoulders. Sit up straight and, ever so slightly, draw the chin in toward the throat. Release any attempt to control the breath or concentrate the mind. Let things go their own way. Simply sit perfectly still, doing nothing at all. Hold this for as long as you like. A regular practice of 20 minutes a day is considered a basic foundation for beginners. For committed meditation practitioners (living a householder's life) 1 to 2 hours per day is considered a sufficient life-long routine.

* **Benefits** Facilitates natural diaphragmatic breathing, aids efficient digestion and assimilation of nutrients, helps the earnest spiritual seeker to embody their Original Nature by releasing striving and attachment; the gesture gives tangible expression to what can't be explained in words.

NOTE If you are sitting in a chair, you can place a shawl or blanket over the lap to give the mudra a more solid foundation to rest on.

DOLA MUDRA
दोलमुद्रा

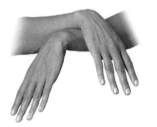

English "swing"

Devanagari दोलमुद्रा

Transliteration Dolamudrā

❋ **Description** *Dola Mudra* is the fifth hand gesture of the twenty-four joint-hand mudras (*samyukta hastas*) as described in the *Abhinaya Darpana*. It is also noted in the *Natya Shastra*. The patron deity associated with it is *Bharati*.

❋ **Technique** There are a few variations regarding the placement of this hand gesture. The basic gesture is depicted as two drooping hands (relaxed wrists), fingers collected and extended, yet relaxed. Make sure to relax your wrists and shoulders while performing this mudra. Variation 1: Placing the relaxed hands on the thighs. Variation 2: Placing each hand by its side of the body. Variation 3: Crossing the hands at the wrists, letting them drop limp across each other.

❋ **Application** Most commonly used at the beginning of a dance piece as an expression of visual eloquence in the pre-dance position. It denotes a "beautiful hand" and adds the quality of grace and femininity (*lasya*) to the presentation of the dancer. This hand can represent infatuation, fainting, drunkenness, intoxication, indolence, excitement, illness, and sadness in the appropriate context.

Dvimukha Mudra

द्विमुखमुद्रा

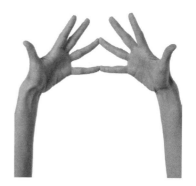

English "two faces"

Devanagari द्विमुखमुद्रा

Transliteration Dvimukhamudrā

❋ **Description** *Dvimukha Mudra* is a joint-hand gesture (*samyukta hasta*) common to the yoga tradition. It is found in the *Yoga Tattva Mudra Vijnana* form, and is one of the traditional thirty-two *Gayatri Mudras*, specifically the fifth gesture in the sub-set of twenty-four mudras practiced before meditation or recitation of the *Gayatri Mantra*.

❋ **Technique** Raise the hands in front of the abdomen, palms facing the midline. Lightly touch the tips of the little and ring fingers of both hands.

❋ **Application** In a comfortable seated position, hold the mudra in front of the abdomen. Breathing naturally, relax the neck, shoulders, and chest. Feel the soothing, sinking quality of Water and the stable, solid quality of Earth. Hold for 5 to 45 minutes.

❋ **Benefits** Balances Water and Earth Elements, benefits the kidneys and improves memory, calms the mind and soothes the belly, activates the body's self-healing capacity, evokes feelings of devotion and purity of heart.

Gada Mudra

गडमुद्रा

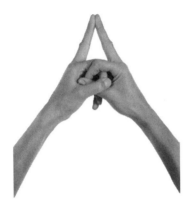

English "mace" or "club"

Devanagari गडमुद्रा

Transliteration Gaḍamudrā

* **Description** *Gada Mudra* is a joint-hand gesture (*samyukta hasta*) used in the Indian Tantric tradition to depict a club or mace. Such a weapon is held by deities to symbolize their fierce commitment to protecting the *Dharma* (spiritual teachings).

* **Technique** Hold the hands in front of you with the palms up. Bend and interlace the little fingers and ring fingers at the second knuckle. Touch the tips of the middle fingers and extend them upward. Then, form two interlocking rings by touching the tips of the index finders and thumbs on both hands.

* **Application** In a comfortable seated position, hold the mudra in front of your pelvis, or in the lap, with the middle fingers pointed forward and slightly up. Relax your belly, breathe naturally, and hold for 5 to 45 minutes.

* **Benefits** Improves elimination and tones the organs of the pelvis, treats hemorrhoids and prolapsed organs, strengthens the *Muladhara Chakra* (root center), opens the flow of rising energy up the back of the body, evokes feelings of stability, groundedness, and safety.

NOTE This mudra may also be used by healing arts practitioners, as a tool to address complaints related to the pelvis and/or feelings of fear or instability. Form the mudra and hold it a few inches above the client's lower belly (about 3 inches below the navel).

GAJADANTA MUDRA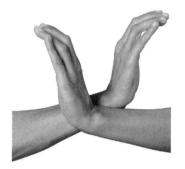

गजदन्तमुद्रा

English "elephant's tusk"

Devanagari गजदन्तमुद्रा

Transliteration Gajadantamudrā

- **Description** *Gajadanta Mudra* is a joint-hand gesture (*samyukta hasta*) noted in the *Natya Shastra* and *Abhinaya Darpana*. The patron deity associated with this mudra is *Paramatma*.[15]

- **Technique** Both hands assume *Sarpashirsha Mudras* (p.213) and are crossed at the forearm, mutually touching the opposite arms between the elbow and the shoulder. (The picture here shows the initial phase of crossing the two hands.)

- **Application** Used by performing artists to denote the following: grasping a pillar, pulling up a stone, carrying the bride and groom on their wedding day, or lifting anything heavy.

GANESHA MUDRA

गणेशमुद्रा

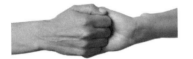

English "remover of obstacles"

Devanagari गणेशमुद्रा

Transliteration Gaṇeśamudrā

* **Description** *Ganesha Mudra* is a joint-hand gesture (*samyukta hasta*) common to the yoga tradition. It is used to evoke the spirit of *Ganesha*, the remover of obstacles, and to generate feelings of stability, confidence, and warmth.

* **Technique** With the left palm facing outward and the right palm facing your chest, bend the fingers to form a "hook" with each hand. Clasp the two hands together and pull gently to create a solid fit.

* **Application** This mudra can be used anytime, while standing, sitting, or walking. For a more concentrated practice, sit in a comfortable position with your spine erect. Roll your shoulders back and down, broaden your chest and back. Hold the mudra in front of your heart for 5 to 20 minutes.

* **Benefits** Opens the chest, facilitates deep breathing, benefits the heart, tones the muscles of the upper back, promotes confidence and courage, evokes the qualities of warmth and care for one's self and others.

GARUDA MUDRA I

गरुडमुद्रा

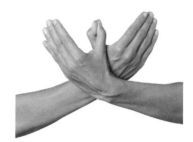

English "mythological bird"

Devanagari गरुडमुद्रा

Transliteration Garuḍamudrā

※ **Description** *Garuda Mudra I* is the twentieth hand gesture of the twenty-four joint-hand mudras (*samyukta hastas*) as described in the *Abhinaya Darpana*.

※ **Technique** Cross the wrists with your hands facing toward your body. Then, interlock the thumbs, keeping your fingers collected. Roll your hands in a wave-like motion to express the movement of a bird's wings in flight.

※ **Application** Denotes an eagle or the mythological bird *Garuda*, who is the vehicle ("*vahanam*") of *Vishnu*.

GARUDA MUDRA II

गरुडमुद्रा

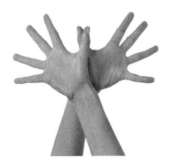

English "mythological bird"

Devanagari गरुडमुद्रा

Transliteration Garuḍamudrā

❋ **Description** *Garuda Mudra II* is a joint-hand gesture (*samyukta hasta*) common in Indian Tantrism and Japanese Buddhism (*Vajrayana*). It depicts a large mythological bird, resembling an eagle. According to tradition, when *Garuda* emerged from his egg he was already fully developed and very powerful. In spiritual parlance, this hints at the notion that our Original Nature is inherently complete, and that enlightenment is not an attainment, but a realization of what is always the case. The image of *Garuda* is a powerful symbol for many cultures throughout Asia. It is found depicted in the military, political, and religious symbolism of Indonesia, Mongolia, India, and Thailand.

❋ **Technique** Raise the hands in front of the chest, palms facing forward. Cross and bend the thumbs, creating a firm pressure between the pads of the fingers. Fan the remaining fingers up and to the sides, in the shape of large wings.

❋ **Application** *Garuda Mudra II* can be used anytime in any position. The mudra has a particular affinity with eagles and other birds of prey, and can be used to connect with the spirit of birds in general while walking or hiking in nature. As a protector, it can be used before a long journey, particularly in the wilderness, that may have unforeseen dangers (especially snakes). For physical health and spiritual cultivation, apply the mudra in a comfortable seated position and visualize yourself as a huge bird soaring high above the ground, observing yourself from above. Continue this practice for 5 to 45 minutes.

❋ **Benefits** Improves intelligence, increases digestive fire, activates *Manipura Chakra* (navel center), builds martial prowess, and, according to legend, serves as protection against snakes, snake bites, and venom in general.

NOTE The image above shows the mudra as seen from the practitioner's view.

GAVAKSHA MUDRA

गवक्षमुद्रा

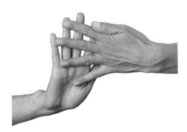

English "air-hole" or "lattice"

Devanagari गवक्षमुद्रा

Transliteration Gavakṣamudrā

⁂ **Description** *Gavaksha Mudra* is a joint-hand gesture (*samyukta hasta*) common to Odissi Dance.

⁂ **Technique** Form *Pataka Mudra* (p.186) with each hand, leaving the fingers slightly separated. Hold the right hand with the palm facing outward, fingers pointing upward at your right side. Place the left hand across the right, palm facing you. The fingers are slightly separated, leaving gaps to peek through.

⁂ **Application** Used by performing artists to express the shyness of the heroine, as she half hides and half peeks through this hand gesture.

NOTE This mudra is very similar to *Chakra Mudra*. The difference is that there are spaces between the fingers, and the placement of the gesture is in front of the face, slightly off to the side.

ग्रन्थितमुद्रा

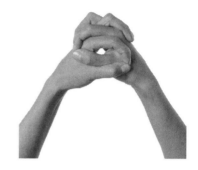

English "knot" or "knot of maya"

Devanagari ग्रन्थितमुद्रा

Transliteration Granthitamudrā

❋ **Description** *Granthita Mudra* is a joint-hand gesture (*samyukta hasta*) common to the yoga tradition. It is found in the *Yoga Tattva Mudra Vijnana* form, and is one of the traditional thirty-two *Gayatri Mudras*, specifically the fourteenth gesture in the sub-set of twenty-four mudras practiced before meditation or recitation of the *Gayatri Mantra*.

❋ **Technique** Clasp the hands together with the left index finger on top of the right. Lightly touch the tips of thumbs and index fingers, forming two rings.

❋ **Application** In a comfortable seated position, hold the mudra in front of the throat. Relax the tongue, jaw, and shoulders. Soften the belly and breathe naturally. Feel the inside of the mouth and throat as a hollow space filled with clear light. Hold for 5 to 45 minutes.

❋ **Benefits** Prepares the mind for meditation, opens *Vishuddha Chakra* (the throat center), benefits the voice, improves thyroid function, increases the body's self-healing capacity, especially in cases of cancer.

GURU MUDRA

गुरुमुद्रा

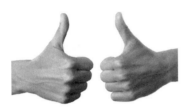

English "planet Jupiter"

Devanagari गुरुमुद्रा

Transliteration Gurumudrā

Additional names *Brhaspati, Dhishana*

⚘ **Description** *Guru Mudra* is a joint-hand gesture (*samyukta hasta*) used by performing artists. It is found in the traditional set of the nine planets (*Nava-Graha Hastas*) as described in the *Abhinaya Darpana*. It indicates the character of the planet Jupiter.

⚘ **Technique** Form *Shikhara Mudra* (p.225) with each hand, as if holding a sacred thread. The gaze is fixed upward.

⚘ **Application** To denote the planet Jupiter. This gesture also indicates a sage (*rishi*) or a *Brahmin* priest.

NOTE Your hands can be held as seen in the image above, or with the left thumb pointing downward by the shoulder and the right thumb pointing upward by the hip.

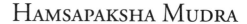

हंसपक्षमुद्रा

English "swan's wing"

Devanagari हंसपक्षमुद्रा

Transliteration Haṁsapakṣamudrā

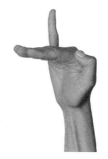

❀ **Description** *Hamsapaksha Mudra* is the twenty-fourth hand gesture of the twenty-eight single-hand mudras (*asamyukta hastas*) as described in the *Abhinaya Darpana*. It is also noted in the *Natya Shastra*. According to mythology, *Tandu* who expounded *Tandava* dance used this gesture while practicing in front of *Shiva*. The associated sage is *Bharata*, race is *Apsara*, color is blue, and patron deity is *Manmatha* (aka *Kamadeva*, the god of love).

❀ **Technique** Hold your hand with the palm facing downward, extend your little finger upward, keeping the index, middle, and little fingers bent at 90 degrees. The tip of the thumb touches the base of the index finger on the outside.

❀ **Application** Primarily used by performing artists to create context and express emotional states or specific actions. *Viniyoga*: *Shat-samkhyam* ("number six"); *Setubandha* ("constructing a bridge"); *Nakha-rekha-ankanam* ("nail marks"); *Pidhana* ("conceal"). Additional usages denote: playing the *veena*,[16] gathering, restraining, bird's wing, completion of work, and drawing a portrait.

Hamsasya Mudra

हंसास्यमुद्रा

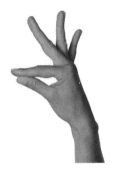

English "swan's face"

Devanagari हंसास्यमुद्रा

Transliteration Haṃsāsyamudrā

- **Description** *Hamsasya Mudra* is the twenty-third hand gesture of the twenty-eight single-hand mudras (*asamyukta hastas*) as described in the *Abhinaya Darpana*. It is also noted in the *Natya Shastra*. According to mythology, this mudra is derived from *Dakshinamurti*[17] when he was explaining the intricacies of the *Tattva* system.[18] Its race is *Brahmin*, and its patron deity is *Brahma*.

- **Technique** Join the tips of the thumb and index finger, keeping both fingers straight and extended. Separate and extend the middle, ring, and little fingers.

- **Application** Primarily used by performing artists to create context and express emotional states or specific actions. *Viniyoga*: *Mangalaye-sutrabandha* ("tying the marriage thread"); *Upadesha* ("initiation" or " instruction"); *Vinischaye* ("certainty"); *Romancha* ("horripilation"); *Mauktika-adau* ("pearl necklace and the like"); *Dipavarti-prasarana* ("extending the wick of a lamp"); *Nikasha* ("touch-stone"); *Mallika-adau* ("Jasmine flower and the like"); *Chithra* ("picture"); *Tat-lekhana* ("drawing a picture"); *Damsha* ("fly bite"); *Jalabhanda* ("drop of water"). Additional usages denote: carrying a garland, metaphor, signifying "I am That" (*so'ham*), accomplishment of a task, ritual, decision, offering, speaking, reading, singing, meditation, smell, taking aim, seal-ring.

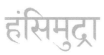

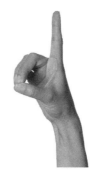

English "containing the spirit"

Devanagari हंसिमुद्रा

Transliteration Haṁsimudrā

* **Description** *Hamsi Mudra* is a single-hand gesture (*asamyukta hasta*) common to the Hindu and yoga traditions. It is found in the *Yoga Tattva Mudra Vijnana* form where it is used to relieve obstacles and restore child-like joy and laughter.

* **Technique** Join the tips of the middle, ring, and little fingers with the tip of the thumb. Extend the index finger.

* **Application** This mudra may be done in any position; while walking, standing, sitting, or reclining. It is best to approach *Hamsi Mudra* with the spirit of play and exploration. Hold as long as you like.

* **Benefits** Removes obstacles in one's life, eases depression and sadness, evokes feelings of lightness and laughter, benefits the lungs and large intestine, improves assimilation of nutrients and elimination of waste.

NOTE In India, *Hamsi Mudra* is commonly practiced along with the recitation of mantras or prayers. It is commonly used during ritual worship, *puja* or *yajna*, to increase the effects of the intended ritual.

Hridaya Mudra

हृदयमुद्रा

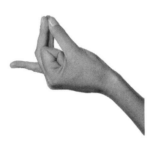

English "heart seal" or "gesture of the heart"

Devanagari हृदयमुद्रा

Transliteration Hṛdayamudrā

* **Description** *Hridaya Mudra* is a single-hand gesture (*asamyukta hasta*) common to the yoga tradition. It is used to strengthen the heart and release pent-up emotions. It is almost identical in appearance and application to *Mritsamjivani Mudra*, with the exception of a subtle, yet important difference in the placement of the index finger.

* **Technique** Roll the index finger down on itself so the tip tucks into the base and the first knuckle touches the base of the thumb. Join the tips of the middle and ring fingers with the thumb. Extend the little finger.

* **Application** May be used anytime in any position to benefit the heart. For more powerful results, form the mudra with each hand and sit quietly in a comfortable position, hands resting palms up on the thighs. Relax the solar plexus (area below the sternum) and breathe naturally. Smile inwardly to your heart, feeling your chest open and relaxed. Hold for 5 to 45 minutes. Practice 2 to 3 sessions per day for best results.

* **Benefits** Rejuvenates the heart and pericardium, releases accumulated stress and emotions, regulates blood pressure and heart rate, reduces anxiety, opens *Anahata Chakra* (heart center).

INDRA MUDRA

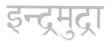

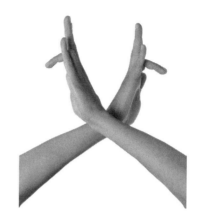

English "deity of heaven and storms"

Devanagari इन्द्रमुद्रा

Transliteration Indramudrā

Additional names *Sakra, Devendra, Devapati*

❋ **Description** *Indra Mudra* is a joint-hand gesture (*samyukta hasta*) used by performing artists. It is found in the traditional set of sixteen *Deva Hastas*, denoting Hindu gods and goddesses as described in the *Abhinaya Darpana*. It indicates the form and character of the Hindu deity *Indra*.

❋ **Technique** Assume *Tripataka Mudra* (p.253) with each hand. Cross the wrists and raise the hands overhead.

❋ **Application** Used to indicate *Indra*, the Hindu god of heaven. Hands are held above the head and symbolize a thunderstorm or mountain.

Jnana Mudra

ज्ञानमुद्रा

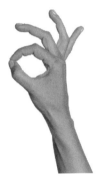

English "seal of wisdom"

Devanagari ज्ञानमुद्रा

Transliteration Jñānamudrā

* **Description** *Jnana Mudra* is the single-hand gesture (*asamyukta hasta*) expressing the "seal of wisdom," common to the yoga tradition. It is found in the *Yoga Tattva Mudra Vijnana* form, and is the most common mudra used for meditation on *pranava*.[19]

* **Technique** Lightly join the tips of the thumb and index finger, with the remaining fingers extended and relaxed.

* **Application** In a comfortable seated position, form the mudra with each hand and place the hands on the knees, palms facing down. Extend the spine, relax the shoulders, and breathe naturally. Lightly focus on the subtle sensations of the physical body. Rest in stillness for 5 to 45 minutes.

* **Benefits** Sharpens the intellect, reduces daydreaming and mental fantasy during meditation, lifts depression, opens the lower lobes of the lungs (especially when accompanied by deep diaphragmatic breathing); centering and grounding.

NOTE *Jnana Mudra* and *Chin Mudra* look identical and are used interchangeably in many schools of yoga. The distinction occurs when the mudra is placed on the thighs or knees during seated meditation practice: palms up, it is referred to as *Chin Mudra;* palms down as *Jnana Mudra.* The former produces a subtle feeling of lightness, while the latter evokes a sense of rootedness.

Jyeshtha Kanishtha Bhratri Mudra

ज्येष्ठकनिष्ठभ्रातृमुद्रा

English "oldest-youngest-brothers"

Devanagari ज्येष्ठकनिष्ठभ्रातृमुद्रा

Transliteration Jyeṣṭhakaniṣṭhabhrātṛmudrā

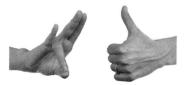

* **Description** *Jyeshtha Kanishtha Bhratri Mudra* is a joint-hand gesture (*samyukta hasta*) used by performing artists. It is found in the traditional set of the eleven relationships (*Bandava Hastas*) as described in the *Abhinaya Darpana.* It indicates brothers.

* **Technique** Assume *Shikhara Mudra* (p.225) with your left hand and *Mayura Mudra* (p.154) with your right hand. Move the hands forward and backward.

* **Application** To denote elder or younger brother.

Kaleshvara Mudra

कालेश्वरमुद्रा

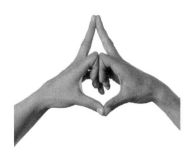

English "lord of time"

Devanagari कालेश्वरमुद्रा

Transliteration Kāleśvaramudrā

❋ **Description** *Kaleshvara Mudra* is a joint-hand gesture (*samyukta hasta*) common to the yoga tradition. It works primarily with the Elements of Fire and Ether, is used to calm the mind, and as a tool to reflect clearly on one's actions.

❋ **Technique** Join the tips of the middle fingers and extend them forward. Fold the index, ring, and little fingers in toward the palms, touching them at the middle joints. Touch the tips of the thumbs together and point them toward the heart.

❋ **Application** In a comfortable seated position, hold the mudra in front of the chest. Drop the shoulders and let the elbows find a natural, relaxed position. Turn your attention inward, allowing the mind to gaze upon itself. Without preference or attachment, simply notice what arises. Hold for 5 to 45 minutes.

❋ **Benefits** Calms and clears the mind, benefits the brain, strengthens the heart and pericardium, assists in the breaking of negative patterns and addictive behaviors.

KAMAJAYI MUDRA

कामजयीमुद्रा

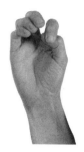

English "conquering lust"

Devanagari कामजयीमुद्रा

Transliteration Kāmajayīmudrā

   ❋   **Description** *Kamajayi Mudra* is a single-hand gesture (*asamyukta hasta*) common to the yoga tradition. It is found in the *Yoga Tattva Mudra Vijnana* form where it is used to subliminate sexual energy into spiritual aspirations.

   ❋   **Technique** Cover the nail of the thumb with the pad of the index finger. The remaining fingers stay relaxed and slightly curled.

   ❋   **Application** This mudra may be done in any position; while walking, standing, sitting, or reclining. It is also effective when applied during practice of yoga *asanas* (postures) where the arms are outstretched.

   ❋   **Benefits** Restrains the outflow of excess passion and sexual desire, causes sexual energy to turn inward and upward (thereby assisting the practice of meditation), strengthens digestion, assimilation, and elimination.

NOTE *Kamajayi Mudra* is traditionally used by celibate yogis while on solitary meditation retreat. It may be employed anytime you wish to temper the flames of sexual desire.

CAUTION Use of this mudra should never be inspired by feelings of guilt or shame around sex or sexuality. A repressive approach to sexual energy can cause serious physiological and psychological problems. Sexual energy is one of the most beautiful and powerful sources of energy in the human body. A balanced and healthy relationship to sexuality is essential for health, longevity, and spiritual growth.

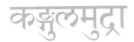

KANGULA MUDRA I

कङ्गुलमुद्रा

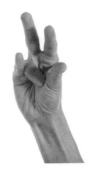

English "tail" or "plough" or "hand"

Devanagari कङ्गुलमुद्रा

Transliteration Kaṅgulamudrā

Additional Name *Langula*

✳ **Description** *Kangula Mudra I* is the nineteenth hand gesture of the twenty-eight single-hand mudras (*asamyukta hastas*) as described in the *Abhinaya Darpana*. It is also noted in the *Natya Shastra*. According to mythology, this mudra derived from *Shiva* when he made a pellet from the poison that sprang from the sea of milk and held it in his hand, forming *Kangula*. The associated sage is *Kumaraswamy*, race is *Siddha*, color is golden, and patron deity is *Lakshmi* or *Padma*.

✳ **Technique** Tuck the ring finger in to the center of the palm and extend the remaining fingers. In a variation of this mudra, the tips of all the remaining fingers touch (see *Kangula Mudra II*).

✳ **Application** Primarily used by performing artists to create context and express emotional states and specific actions. *Viniyoga*: *Lakuchasyapala* ("lakucha fruit"); *Bala-kucha* ("young girl's breast"); *Kalharaka* ("white water-lily"); *Chakora* ("partridge"); *Kramuka* ("betel-nut tree"); *Bala-kimkinyam* ("baby's anklets"); *Ghutika-adika* ("pill"); *Chataka* ("chataka bird"); *Nalikera* ("coconut"); *Gantika* ("bell"). Additional usages denote: grapes, *rudraksha* seed, holding the chin, nipples, star, balls of snow, jasmine flowers, and any small object.

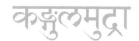

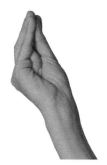

English "tail" or "plough" or "hand"

Devanagari कङ्गुलमुद्रा

Transliteration Kaṅgulamudrā

❋ **Description** *Kangula Mudra II* is a single-hand gesture (*asamyukta hasta*) used in the Hindu tradition to represent a nut, seed, or anything that is small yet contains great potential. By forming the mudra, the ring finger (Earth) is contained and concealed by all the other fingers and Elements. This is symbolic of the hidden power of the human spirit.

❋ **Technique** Curl the ring finger down into the palm. Join the tips of the index, middle, and little finger together with the thumb.

❋ **Application** In a comfortable seated position, form the mudra with each hand and place the hands on the thighs, palms up. Gather the saliva in your mouth and swallow it in three gulps. Feel the saliva travel all the way to your navel, as if you were swallowing seeds of light. Then, soften your belly and chest and breathe naturally. Rest your attention lightly on the sensation at your navel center. Hold for 5 to 45 minutes.

❋ **Benefits** Improves digestion and assimilation, activates hidden talents and gifts, awakens somatic intuition (gut feeling), harmonizes human biorhythms with the rhythms and cycles of the Earth.

NOTE When endeavoring to activate hidden potential within ourselves, it is important to always cultivate a virtuous foundation first. The most foolproof way of doing this is thinking of how we can use our talents to benefit all beings. Here is a simple prayer you can use for this purpose: "May my thoughts, words, and actions be in alignment with the highest good for all beings."

Kapittha Mudra I

कपित्थमुद्रा

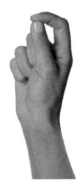

English "wood-apple"

Devanagari कपित्थमुद्रा

Transliteration Kapitthamudrā

Additional Name *Ankusha*

* **Description** *Kapittha Mudra I* is the eleventh hand gesture of the twenty-eight single-hand mudras (*asamyukta hastas*) as described in the *Abhinaya Darpana*. It is also noted in the *Natya Shastra*, and in the *Abhinaya Chandrika* (as *Ankusha*). According to mythology, this mudra originates from the time gods completed churning the ocean of milk to release the nectar of immortality. *Vishnu* then used this hand gesture to pull Mount Mandara from the waters. The associated sage is *Narada*, race is *Rishi*, color is smoky-white, and patron deity is *Padmagarbha* (*Vishnu*).

* **Technique** Tuck the little, ring, and middle fingers into the palm. Extend the thumb straight up, placing the pad of the index finger on the tip of the thumb.

* **Application** Primarily used by performing artists to create context and express emotional states or specific actions. *Viniyoga*: *Lakshmyam* ("Goddess Lakshmi"); *Sarasvatyam* ("Goddess Sarasvati"); *Veshtane* ("winding"); *Taladharana* ("holding cymbals"); *Godohanam* ("milking cows"); *Anjanam* ("applying collyrium"); *Lilakusuma-dharana* ("holding flowers gracefully"); *Chelanchala-adi-grahana* ("grasping the end of a *saree* or a robe"); *Patasya-iva-avaguntana* ("covering the head with a veil"); *Dhupa-dipa-archanam* ("offering incense").

कपित्थमुद्रा

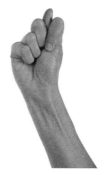

English "elephant apple" or "wood apple"

Devanagari कपित्थमुद्रा

Transliteration Kapitthamudrā

❋ **Description** *Kapittha Mudra II* is a single-hand gesture (*asamyukta hasta*) common to the Hindu tradition. It is usually seen depicted by a deity, and represents the ritual offering of incense or fruit (specifically a wood apple), the female sexual organ, and the act of sexual union.

❋ **Technique** Insert the thumb in the web between the index and middle fingers. Close all the remaining fingers as if making a fist.

❋ **Application** In a comfortable seated position, form the mudra with each hand. Place the left hand against the heart, and the right hand against the pubic bone. Soften the chest, throat, and belly, and breathe naturally. Focus on the feeling of unity between the sexual and spiritual aspects of your life. Hold for 5 to 45 minutes.

❋ **Benefits** Can be used as a tool for sexual healing (releasing guilt and shame around sexuality), increases sensitivity and receptivity, stimulates healthy libido, opens the connection between the pelvis and heart, expands feelings of devotion and loving kindness.

KAPOTA MUDRA
कपोतमुद्रा

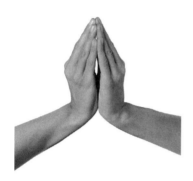

English "dove"

Devanagari कपोतमुद्रा

Transliteration Kapotamudrā

⬥ **Description** *Kapota Mudra* is the second hand gesture of the twenty-four joint-hand mudras (*samyukta hastas*) as described in the *Abhinaya Darpana*. It is also noted in the *Natya Shastra* and *Abhinaya Chandrika*. The patron deity associated with it is *Chitrasena*.

⬥ **Technique** Join the hands palm to palm, as in *Anjali Mudra* (p.44), and create a hollow space between your palms by cupping them away from each other.

⬥ **Application** Primarily used by performing artists to create context and express emotional states or specific actions. *Viniyoga*: *Praname* ("bowing" or "taking oath"); *Guru-sambhasha* ("conversation with teachers or elders"); *Vinaya-angikritishu* ("agreeing humbly"). Additional usages according to the *Natya Shastra*: acquiescence, rows of trees, plantain flower, cold, modesty, collecting things, citron, and casket.

⬥ **Benefits** Used to cultivate humbleness and inward reflection. Can be used to dispel anxiety and coldness by separating the hands quickly and repeatedly forming the gesture.

करग्रमिलितमुद्रा

English "fingertips joined"

Devanagari करग्रमिलितमुद्रा

Transliteration Karagramilitamudrā

Additional Name *Lata*

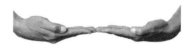

◈ **Description** *Karagra Milita Mudra* is a joint-hand gesture (*samyutka hasta*) mentioned in the *Odissi Dance Pathfinder Vol. II*. An identical mudra named *Lata* ("creeper") is mentioned in several ancient texts such as the *Abhinaya Darpana* and the *Natya Shastra*. The patron deity associated is *Shakti*.

◈ **Technique** Place your hands about 6 inches in front of your navel, with the palms face up and middle fingers touching at the tips. Keep your shoulders relaxed and arms slightly rounded.

◈ **Application** Used at the beginning of a type of ancient South Indian dance called *Svabhava Natana* ("spontaneous pure dance"). Denotes swing, motionless, "heavy with drink," lines, and union. This mudra is often used in Classical Indian Dance to initiate a graceful "pure dance" movement.

KARANA MUDRA

करणमुद्रा

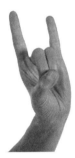

English "of the senses," "the cause," "the reason," or "an instrument"

Devanagari करणमुद्रा

Transliteration Karaṇamudrā

❋ **Description** *Karana Mudra* is a single-hand gesture (*asamyukta hasta*) used in Indian Tantrism and *Vajrayana* (Tantric) Buddhism. It is employed as a ritual instrument to cast out demons and protect the *Dharma* against corruption. It is similar in appearance to the *Venu Mudra* (p.277), and may also be used in Indian dance to depict the drum held by *Shiva Nataraja* or the flute held by Lord *Krishna*.

❋ **Technique** With the pad of the thumb, cover the tips of the middle and ring fingers. Extend the index and little fingers.

❋ **Application** For physical and mental benefits, sit in a comfortable position with the spine erect. Form the mudra with each hand, resting the hands on the lap, palms up. Breathe naturally, and hold for 5 to 45 minutes.

❋ **Benefits** Cleansing and purifying, benefits the bladder, colon, and large intestine, detoxifies body and mind, assists with the release of negative patterns and habits.

NOTE For clearing space or cleansing a room of unwanted energies, form *Karana Mudra* with the right hand and *Kashyapa Mudra* (p.119) with the left hand. Hold *Karana Mudra* firmly against the small of your lower back, and use *Karana Mudra* in front of you, similar to the way you might use a bundle of dried sage to clean and clear the space of unwanted energies. Conclude by opening all the doors and windows, lighting incense, and filling the space with sacred sound (ringing a bell or Tibetan bowl, or chanting HONG loudly).

Karatala Milita Mudra
करतलमिलितमुद्रा

English "hand-palms joined"

Devanagari करतलमिलितमुद्रा

Transliteration Karatalamilitamudrā

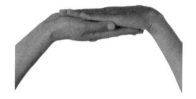

❋ **Description** *Karatala Milita Mudra* is a joint-hand gesture (*samyukta hasta*) mentioned in the *Odissi Dance Pathfinder Vol. II*. It is used mostly in *Pallavis*.[20]

❋ **Technique** Join the hands palm to palm, with fingertips facing opposite directions.

❋ **Application** Held above the head, to frame the face and highlight expression, or in front of the waistline, to draw attention to the feminine curvature of the dancer's figure.

KARKATA MUDRA

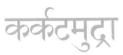
कर्कटमुद्रा

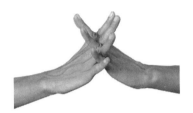

English "crab"

Devanagari कर्कटमुद्रा

Transliteration Karkaṭamudrā

Additional names *Lina Karata, Badha*

❋ **Description** *Karkata Mudra* is the third hand gesture of the twenty-four joint-hand mudras (*samyukta hastas*) as described in the *Abhinaya Darpana*. It is also noted in the *Natya Shastra*. The patron deity associated is *Vishnu*.

❋ **Technique** Extend and interlock the fingers of both hands, maintaining ample space between the palms.

❋ **Application** Primarily used by performing artists to create context and express emotional states or specific actions. *Viniyoga*: *Samuha-agamane* ("arrival of a group" or "coming together as a group"); *Tunda-darshana* ("stomach" or "stout"); *Shanka-purana* ("blowing the conch"); *Anganam-mootana* ("limbs stretching" or "fingers cracking"); *Shakha-unamana* ("bending a branch"). Additional usages denote: lamentation, yawning, striking, breathing hard, and crab.

कर्कटिकमुद्रा

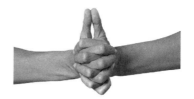

English "kernel"

Devanagari कर्कटिकमुद्रा

Transliteration Karkaṭikamudrā

❋ **Description** *Karkatika Mudra* is a joint-hand gesture (*samyukta hasta*) noted in the *Abhinaya Chandrika.*

❋ **Technique** Interlace the fingers and clasp the hands. Extend the thumbs upward. Stretch your arms forward, keeping the mudra in front of your torso.

❋ **Application** Commonly held during dance conditioning exercises to help develop strength and focus.

❋ **Benefits** Aids in the development of strength, stamina, and concentration.

KARTARIDANDA MUDRA
कर्तरिदण्डमुद्रा

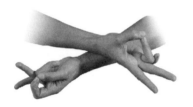

English "arrow shaft"

Devanagari कर्तरिदण्डमुद्रा

Transliteration Kartaridaṇḍamudrā

❋ **Description** *Kartaridanda Mudra* is a joint-hand gesture (*samyukta hasta*) common to the dance tradition. In the *Abhinaya Darpana,* it is noted as one of the gestures that indicate "water animals."

❋ **Technique** Assume *Kartarimukha Mudra I* (p.115) with your right hand and *Katakamukha Mudra III* (p.122) with your left hand. Cross the right forearm on top of the left, and turn both palms to face up.

❋ **Application** Denotes a water snake (*dundubha*).

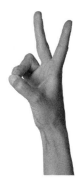

कर्तरिमुखमुद्रा

English "arrow face"

Devanagari कर्तरिमुखमुद्रा

Transliteration Kartarimukhamudrā

❋ **Description** *Kartarimukha Mudra I* is the fourth hand gesture of the twenty-eight single-hand mudras (*asamyukta hastas*) as described in the *Abhinaya Darpana*. It is also noted in *Natya Shastra* and *Abhinaya Chandrika*. According to mythology, this mudra originated from *Shiva* when he set out to slay the demon *Jatadhara*. According to legend, he fixed his middle finger in the center of the earth and drew a circle around the circumference of the earth with his index finger, and this is how *Kartarimukha Mudra* was created. The associated sage is *Parjanya* ("rain god"), race is *Kshatriya*, color is copper, and patron deity is *Vishnu*.

❋ **Technique** Raise your hand with the palm facing forward, fingers pointing upward. Separate the index and middle fingers into a scissor-like shape. Join the tips of the thumb with the tips of the ring and little finger.

❋ **Application** Primarily used by performing artists to create context and express emotional states or specific actions. *Viniyoga: Stri-pumsayu-vishlasya* ("separation of man and woman"); *Viparyasapaday-piva* ("opposition" or "overturning"); *Luntana* ("stealing" or "rolling"); *Nayana-amtam* ("corner of the eye"); *Marana* ("death"); *Bheda-bhavana* ("disagreement"); *Vidhyu-dartha* ("lightning"); *Yekashiya-viraha* ("laying in separation from the loved one"); *Patana* ("falling"); *Latayan* ("creeper"). According to the *Natya Shastra*, when the fingers are pointing downward it can indicate walking, painting the feet, decorating the body, and dancing. When the fingers point upward it can represent biting, blowing a horn, or painting a picture. Additional usages are: lightning, buffalo, deer, flywhisk, hilltop, elephant, bull, cow, coil of hair, scissors, tower.

NOTE In the *Hasta Lakshana Deepika*, this mudra is described as a different formation, similar to *Chatura Mudra* of *Abhinaya Darpana* and *Natya Shastra*.

KARTARIMUKHA MUDRA II

कर्तरिमुखमुद्रा

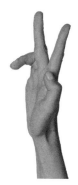

English "arrow face"

Devanagari कर्तरिमुखमुद्रा

Transliteration Kartarimukhamudrā

   ❋   **Description** *Kartarimukha Mudra II* is the fourth hand gesture of the twenty-eight single-hand mudras (*asamyukta hastas*) as described in the *Abhinaya Darpana*. According to mythology, this mudra originated from *Shiva* when he set out to slay the demon *Jatadhara*. According to legend, he fixed his middle finger in the center of the earth and drew a circle around the circumference of the earth with his index finger, and this is how *Kartarimukha Mudra* was created. The associated sage is *Parjanya* ("rain god"), race is *Kshatriya*, color is copper, and patron deity is *Vishnu*.

   ❋   **Technique** Raise your hand with the palm facing forward, fingers pointing upward. Bend the little and ring fingers 90 degrees at the lower joint. Separate the index and middle fingers into a scissor-like shape. Keep the thumb flush against the side of the hand.

   ❋   **Application** See *Kartarimukha Mudra I*.

NOTE Another variation, mentioned in the *Odissi Dance Pathfinder*,[21] is with fingers and thumb extended upward; bend the middle and ring fingers deep toward the palm.

KARTARISVASTIKA MUDRA
कर्तरिस्वस्तिकमुद्रा

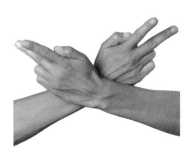

English "crossed arrows"

Devanagari कर्तरिस्वस्तिकमुद्रा

Transliteration Kartarisvastikamudrā

* **Description** *Kartarisvastika Mudra* is the tenth hand gesture of the twenty-four joint-hand mudras (*samyukta hastas*) as described in the *Abhinaya Darpana*.

* **Technique** Form *Kartarimukha Mudra I* or *II* (p.115/p.117) with each hand. Cross the wrists and keep the gesture about 6 inches from your chest.

* **Application** Primarily used by performing artists to create context and express emotional states or specific actions. *Viniyoga*: *Shakha* ("branches of a tree"); *Adri-Shikara* ("summit or hill top"); *Vriksha* ("tree").

NOTE This mudra is also noted in the *Abhinaya Darpana* as describing a specific type of tree named *Shami*.

कश्यपमुद्रा

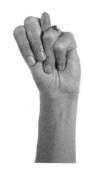

English "turtle/tortoise gesture"

Devanagari कश्यपमुद्रा

Transliteration Kaśyapamudrā

❋ **Description** *Kashyapa Mudra* is a single-hand gesture (*asamyukta hasta*) used in the Hindu tradition to depict the union of *linga* and *yoni,* and to symbolize *Kashyapa Rishi.*[22]

❋ **Technique** Place the tip of the thumb in the web between the middle and ring fingers. Close the remaining fingers as if making a fist.

❋ **Application** In a comfortable seated position, form the mudra with each hand and place the hands on the thighs, palms facing up. Relax the throat, chest, and belly. Breathe naturally and hold for 5 to 45 minutes.

❋ **Benefits** Grounding and centering, balances masculine and feminine qualities, protects against negative energies and unfriendly or confused spirits (sometimes called "orphan spirits").

NOTE *Kashyapa Mudra* can also be used as a protective seal placed in the small of the lower back during energetic purification of a room or building (a practice similar to what is commonly called "smudging" in Native American traditions). In this case, the mudra is formed with the left hand while the right holds a stick of incense or bundle of dried sage.

KATAKAMUKHA MUDRA I

कटकमुखमुद्रा

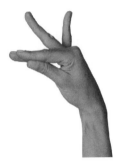

English "link in a chain"

Devanagari कटकमुखमुद्रा

Transliteration Kaṭakamukhamudrā

* **Description** *Katakamukha Mudra I* is the twelfth hand gesture of the twenty-eight single-hand mudras (*asamyukta hastas*) as described in the *Abhinaya Darpana*. According to mythology, this mudra originated from *Guha*[23] when he practiced archery in front of *Shiva*. The associated sage is *Bhargava*, race is *Deva*, color is gold, and patron deity is *Raghu Rama*.

* **Technique** Join the tip of the thumb, index, and middle fingers. Keep these fingers extended and active. Stretch the ring and little fingers upward.

* **Application** Primarily used by performing artists to create context and express emotional states or specific actions. It is one of the most common mudras used in *Pallavis* ("pure dance"). *Viniyoga*: *Kusuma-apachaye* ("plucking flowers"); *Mukta-srak-damnam-dharanam* ("wearing a necklace of pearls or flowers"); *Nagavalli-pradhanam* ("offering betel leaves"); *Kasturika-adivastunam-peshana* ("preparing paste for musk, etc."); *Gandhavasana* ("to smell"); *Vachana* ("to speak"); *Drishti* ("glancing").

KATAKAMUKHA MUDRA II

कटकमुखमुद्रा

English "link in a chain"

Devanagari कटकमुखमुद्रा

Transliteration Kaṭakamukhamudrā

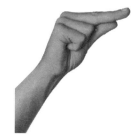

❋ **Description** *Katakamukha Mudra II* is the twelfth hand gesture of the twenty-eight single-hand mudras (*asamyukta hastas*) as described in the *Abhinaya Darpana*. According to mythology, this mudra originated from *Guha* when he practiced archery in front of *Shiva*. The associated sage is *Bhargava*, race is *Deva*, color is gold, and patron deity is *Raghu Rama*.

❋ **Technique** Join the tip of the thumb, index, and middle finger, keeping them extended and active. Tuck the ring and little finger into the palm.

❋ **Application** See *Katakamukha Mudra I*.

NOTE This version is mentioned in the *Odissi Dance Pathfinder Vol. I.*[24]

Katakamukha Mudra III

कटकमुखमुद्रा

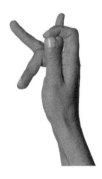

English "link in a chain"

Devanagari कटकमुखमुद्रा

Transliteration Kaṭakamukhamudrā

* **Description** *Katakamukha Mudra III* is a single-hand gesture (*asamyukta hasta*) noted in the *Natya Shastra*. Like *Katakamukha Mudra I*, it is often used in *Pallavis* ("pure dance").

* **Technique** Straighten the thumb and place the pad of the index finger on top of it. Point the middle finger downward, and stretch the ring and little fingers upward.

* **Application** *Sara-madhya-akarshanam* ("drawing the arrow in the center of the bow"); holding a mirror, fanning, holding reins, breaking a twig, cleaning the teeth, plucking flowers, embracing, holding a disc, pulling a rope, and tucking or holding the loose end of a veil or a robe.

KATAKAVARDHANA MUDRA

कटकवर्धनमुद्रा

English "link of increase"

Devanagari कटकवर्धनमुद्रा

Transliteration Kaṭakavardhanamudrā

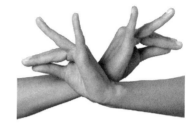

❋ **Description** *Katakavardhana Mudra* is the ninth hand gesture of the twenty-four joint-hand mudras (*samyukta hastas*) as described in the *Abhinaya Darpana*. It is also noted in the *Natya Shastra*. The patron deity associated with it is *Yaksharaja*.[25]

❋ **Technique** Form *Katakamukha Mudra I* (p.115) with each hand and cross at the wrists. Keep the gesture a hand's distance away from your body.

❋ **Application** Primarily used by performing artists to create context and express emotional states or specific actions. *Viniyoga: Pattabhisheke* ("coronation"); *Pujayam* ("ritual"); *Vivaha-ashishi* ("marriage blessings"). Additional usages denote: deliberation, erotic mood, pacification, certainty, and the dances known as *Jakkini-natana* and *Danda-lasya*.

Ketaki Mudra
केतकीमुद्रा

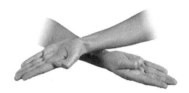

English "screw-pine tree"

Devanagari केतकीमुद्रा

Transliteration Ketakīmudrā

❋ **Description** *Ketaki Mudra* is a joint-hand gesture (*samyukta hasta*) common to the dance tradition. In the *Abhinaya Darpana*, it is noted as one of the gestures that indicate "trees."

❋ **Technique** Assume *Pataka Mudra* (p.186) with your left hand and *Chatura Mudra* (p.73) with your right hand. Cross the wrists and turn both palms to face upward.

❋ **Application** Used in the dance tradition to denote the flower of the screw-pine tree.

केतुमुद्रा

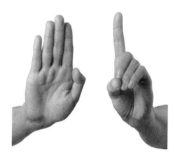

English "dragon's tail"

Devanagari केतुमुद्रा

Transliteration Ketumudrā

❋ **Description** *Ketu Mudra* is a joint-hand gesture (*samyukta hasta*) used by performing artists. It is found in the traditional set of the nine planets (*Nava-Graha Hastas*) as described in the *Abhinaya Darpana*. In Vedic astrology, *Ketu* is the Moon's south (descending) node. *Ketu* is generally referred to as a "shadow" planet.

❋ **Technique** Assume *Suchi Mudra* (p.240) with your left hand and *Pataka Mudra* (p.186) with your right hand. Place your hands in front of your chest. Evoke a cruel gaze and mood.

❋ **Application** To denote the descending (south) lunar node, *Ketu*.

Khatva Mudra

खत्वामुद्रा

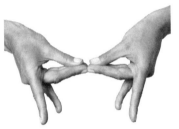

English "cot"

Devanagari खत्वामुद्रा

Transliteration Khaṭvāmudrā

* **Description** *Khatva Mudra* is the twenty-second hand gesture of the twenty-four joint-hand mudras (*samyukta hastas*) as described in the *Abhinaya Darpana.*

* **Technique** Join the pad of the thumb with the pads of the middle and ring fingers. Connect the two hands by joining the tips of thumbs, middle, and ring fingers at the center. Turn the hands palms up and extend the index and little fingers downward like the legs of a bed or cot. Hold the mudra at hip height.

* **Application** Used to denote a cot, a bed, or a bench. In dance, it is often used to show the sitting place of the various deities.

NOTE In a variation of this mudra, the tips of the thumbs touch the base of the middle and ring fingers.

किलकमुद्रा

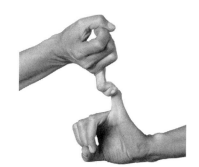

English "bond"

Devanagari किलकमुद्रा

Transliteration Kilakamudrā

* **Description** *Kilaka Mudra I* is the sixteenth hand gesture of the twenty-four joint-hand mudras (*samyukta hastas*) as described in the *Abhinaya Darpana*.

* **Technique** With each hand, fold the index, middle, and ring fingers into the palm and place the thumb on top. Interlock the little fingers at the top joint.

* **Application** Primarily used by performing artists to create context and express emotional states or specific actions. *Viniyoga*: *Snehe* ("affection," or "in love"); *Narmanulapa* ("lovers' conversation").

KILAKA MUDRA II
किलकमुद्रा

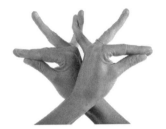

English "bond"

Devanagari किलकमुद्रा

Transliteration Kilakamudrā

❋ **Description** *Kilaka Mudra II* is a joint-hand mudra (*samyukta hasta*) commonly used to indicate the energy of intimacy and amorous relations. The version presented here is more commonly seen in the context of Japanese Tantric Buddhism.

❋ **Technique** Cross the wrists with the hands back to back. Hook the little fingers with the tips pointing upward. Join the thumb, index, and middle finger on each hand. Extend the ring fingers upward at about a 45-degree angle.

❋ **Application** In a comfortable seated position, hold the mudra in front of the heart a comfortable distance from the body. Relax the throat, chest, and belly. Breathe naturally and hold for 5 to 45 minutes.

❋ **Benefits** Tonifies the Water Element in the body, improves the function of the kidneys, bladder, and sexual glands, fosters a sense of emotional safety and comfort around intimacy and sexuality, can also be used as a devotional gesture to express or evoke the union of masculine (*Shiva*) and feminine (*Shakti*).[26]

किरीटमुद्रा

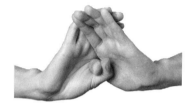

English "crown"

Devanagari किरीटमुद्रा

Transliteration Kirīṭamudrā

- ❋ **Description** *Kirita Mudra* is a joint-hand gesture (*samyukta hasta*) common to the dance tradition.

- ❋ **Technique** With both palms facing forward, connect the pads of the thumbs. The fingers of one hand will cover those of the other.

- ❋ **Application** Used in the dance tradition to denote a crown (or a king) when placed above the head.

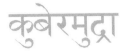

KUBERA MUDRA I

कुबेरमुद्रा

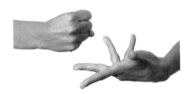

English "god of wealth"

Devanagari कुबेरमुद्रा

Transliteration Kuberamudrā

🏵 **Description** *Kubera Mudra I* is a joint-hand gesture (*samyukta hasta*) used by performing artists. It is found in the traditional set of sixteen *Deva Hastas*, denoting Hindu gods and goddesses as described in the *Abhinaya Darpana*. It indicates the form and character of the Hindu deity *Kubera*.

🏵 **Technique** Assume *Alapadma Mudra* (p.41) with your left hand and *Mushti Mudra* (p.163) with your right hand. Hold your hands about 6 inches in front of your body.

🏵 **Application** Used to indicate *Kubera*, the Hindu god of wealth.

NOTE There are several combinations of mudras used to express the various traits and emblems of *Kubera Deva*. The gesture indicated here appears to be the most common.

कुबेरमुद्रा

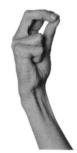

English "god of wealth"

Devanagari कुबेरमुद्रा

Transliteration Kuberamudrā

⁕ **Description** *Kubera Mudra II* is a single-hand gesture (*asamyukta hasta*) common to the Hindu tradition. It is used to create abundance, to evoke blessings from the "god of wealth," and to symbolize the northern direction. *Kubera* is known in the Buddhist tradition as *Vaishravana*, chief of the Four Heavenly Kings.

⁕ **Technique** Join the tips of the thumb, index, and middle finger. Curl the ring and little fingers into the palm.

⁕ **Application** In a comfortable seated position, form the mudra with each hand, resting the hands in your lap, palms up. Soften the belly and breathe naturally. Focus on what you would like to attract more of in your life. Feel the mudra serving as a magnet, helping you manifest your desires. Hold for 5 to 45 minutes.

⁕ **Benefits** Clears the frontal sinuses and helps to balance left and right nostrils, improves sense of smell, sharpens "inner vision" and ability to more clearly see your path in life, helps create abundance, especially related to virtuous desires that take into consideration the welfare of all beings.

KURMA MUDRA I

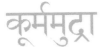

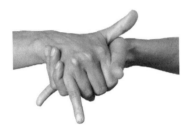

English "tortoise"

Devanagari कूर्ममुद्रा

Transliteration Kūrmamudrā

- **Description** *Kurma Mudra I* is the eighteenth hand gesture of the twenty-four joint-hand mudras (*samyukta hastas*) as described in the *Abhinaya Darpana*.

- **Technique** With the hands touching palm to palm, fold the index, middle, and ring fingers of both hands over the other, keeping the little fingers and thumbs extended.

- **Application** Denotes a tortoise, known in Hindu mythology as the second incarnation ("*avatara*") of *Vishnu*. To convey the movement of the tortoise, move your wrists back and forth.

KURMA MUDRA II

कूर्ममुद्रा

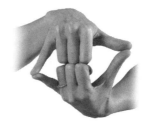

English "tortoise"

Devanagari कूर्ममुद्रा

Transliteration Kūrmamudrā

❋ **Description** *Kurma Mudra II* is a less common variation of the eighteenth hand gesture of the twenty-four joint-hand mudras (*samyukta hastas*) as described in the *Abhinaya Darpana*.

❋ **Technique** With each hand, fold the index, middle, and ring fingers into the palm. Extend the thumbs and little fingers away from each other. Join the two hands together as mirror images with the right on top of the left. The tips of the little fingers and thumbs touch, and the knuckles press together firmly.

❋ **Application** See *Kurma Mudra I*.

KURMA MUDRA III
कूर्ममुद्रा

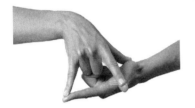

English "tortoise"

Devanagari कूर्ममुद्रा

Transliteration Kūrmamudrā

❋ **Description** *Kurma Mudra III* is a joint-hand gesture (*samyukta hasta*) common to the yoga tradition where it represents one of the auspicious forms *Vishnu* assumed to benefit humanity. It is found in the *Yoga Tattva Mudra Vijnana* form, and is one of the traditional thirty-two *Gayatri Mudras*, specifically the nineteenth gesture in the sub-set of twenty-four mudras practiced before meditation or recitation of the *Gayatri Mantra*. The mudra is unique energetically in that it forms a triangular relationship between Air, Water, and Fire Elements, which serves to harmonize *ojas*, *tejas*, and *prana* in the body (see Appendix A).

❋ **Technique** Turn the left palm up, folding the middle, ring, and little fingers into the palm. Extend the thumb and index finger. Turn the right palm down, folding the middle and ring fingers into the palm. Extend the thumb, index, and little finger. Rest the right hand on top of the left. Join the right index with the left thumb, and the right little finger with the left index. The right thumb rests against the base of the left thumb, near the wrist.

❋ **Application** In a comfortable seated position, hold the mudra in front of your solar plexus (below the sternum). Soften your belly, chest, and shoulders. Breathe naturally, settling into relaxed stillness. Hold for 5 to 45 minutes.

❋ **Benefits** Activates the body's self-healing power, balances the immune system (reducing the negative effects of hypo- or hyper-immunity), harmonizes the relationship between the heart (Fire) and the kidneys (Water).

NOTE According to the yogic tradition, it is said that *Kurma Mudra* can be used for assisting the healing of major diseases, especially cancer.

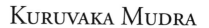

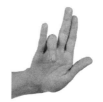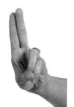

English "henna plant"

Devanagari कुरुवकमुद्रा

Transliteration Kuruvakamudrā

❋ **Description** *Kuruvaka Mudra* is a joint-hand gesture (*samyukta hasta*) common to the dance tradition. In the *Abhinaya Darpana*, it is noted as one of the gestures that indicate "trees."

❋ **Technique** Assume *Tripataka Mudra* (p.253) with your right hand and *Kartarimukha Mudra I* (p.115) with your left hand. Both hands are held in front of the chest, palms facing outward.

❋ **Application** Used in the dance tradition to denote the henna plant.

LAKSHMI MUDRA
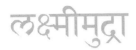

English "goddess of fortune, wealth, and grace"

Devanagari लक्ष्मीमुद्रा

Transliteration Lakṣmīmudrā

Additional Name *Mahalakshmi*

❋ **Description** *Lakshmi Mudra* is a joint-hand gesture (*samyukta hasta*) used by performing artists. It is found in the traditional set of sixteen *Deva Hastas*, denoting Hindu gods and goddesses as described in the *Abhinaya Darpana*. It indicates the form and character of the Hindu deity *Lakshmi*.

❋ **Technique** Form *Kapittha Mudra* (p.106) with each hand, holding the hands near the shoulders.

❋ **Application** Used to indicate *Lakshmi*, the Hindu goddess of wealth, prosperity (both material and spiritual), light, wisdom, fortune, fertility, generosity, and courage; and the embodiment of beauty, grace, and charm. She is the consort of *Vishnu*.

NOTE There are several combinations of mudras used to express the various traits and emblems of *Lakshmi Devi*. The gesture indicated here appears to be the most common.

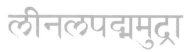

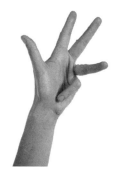

English "bees clinging to the lotus flower"

Devanagari लीनलपद्ममुद्रा

Transliteration Līnalapadmamudrā

❋ **Description** *Linalapadma Mudra* is a single-hand gesture (*asamyukta hasta*) common to the dance tradition. In the *Abhinaya Darpana*, it is noted as one of the gestures that indicate "flying creatures."

❋ **Technique** Touch the tip of the little finger to the palm. Extend the thumb and remaining fingers outward and maintain space between them.

❋ **Application** Used in the dance tradition to denote the curlew bird, or a blossoming flower attracting bees.

NOTE This mudra is similar to *Alapadma* and *Baka*.

LINGA MUDRA
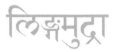
लिङ्गमुद्रा

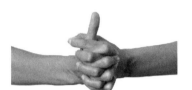

English "phallus," "divine masculine," or "cosmic consciousness"

Devanagari लिङ्गमुद्रा

Transliteration Liṅgamudrā

❋ **Description** *Linga Mudra* is a joint-hand gesture (*samyukta hasta*) common to the yoga tradition. It is found in the *Yoga Tattva Mudra Vijnana* form, and is one of the traditional thirty-two *Gayatri Mudras*, specifically the seventh gesture in the sub-set of eight mudras practiced after meditation or recitation of the *Gayatri Mantra*.

❋ **Technique** Interlock the fingers of both hands with the left index finger on top. Extend the right thumb straight up. Join the tips of the left thumb and index finger, forming a circle around the extended thumb.

❋ **Application** In a comfortable seated position, hold the mudra in front of the abdomen. Relax the chest, belly, and throat. Breathe naturally. Hold for 5 to 45 minutes.

❋ **Benefits** Warms the body, relieves cold and flu symptoms, reduces lethargy and laziness, increases self-confidence and willpower.

लोलितमुद्रा

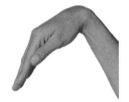

English "moved hither and thither"

Devanagari लोलितमुद्रा

Transliteration Lolitamudrā

* **Description** *Lolita Mudra* is a single-hand gesture (*asamyukta hasta*) noted in the *Abhinaya Chandrika*. It is similar to *Dola Mudra* but performed with a single hand rather than two hands.

* **Technique** Relax your wrist, letting the hand drop. The hand sways gently resembling a swing with the movement of walking or dancing.

* **Application** Used to denote the graceful movement of women. Expresses grace, beauty, young women, etc. To accentuate the grace and sensual nuance of *Pallavi*s ("pure form") dances, the performer will often use *Lolita Mudra* while depicting a female character. Often held low by one's side while relaxing the shoulder and arm.

MADHYAPATAKA MUDRA

मध्यपताकमुद्रा

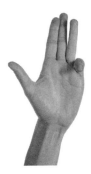

English "middle flag"

Devanagari मध्यपताकमुद्रा

Transliteration Madhyapatākamudrā

❋ **Description** *Madhyapataka Mudra* is a single-hand gesture (*asamyukta hasta*) common to the dance tradition. In the *Abhinaya Darpana*, it is noted as one of the gestures that indicate "wild animals."

❋ **Technique** Fold the little finger toward the palm and extend the remaining fingers upward.

❋ **Application** Used in the dance tradition to denote a dog. When used with both hands connected at the wrist, this mudra denotes the open mouth of a crocodile.

महाक्रान्तमुद्रा

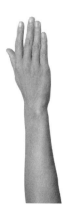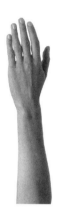

English "supreme power"

Devanagari महाक्रान्तमुद्रा

Transliteration Mahākrāntamudrā

* **Description** *Mahakranta Mudra* is a joint-hand gesture (*samyukta hasta*) common to the yoga tradition. It is found in the *Yoga Tattva Mudra Vijnana* form, and is one of the traditional thirty-two *Gayatri Mudras*, specifically the twenty-second gesture in the sub-set of twenty-four mudras practiced before meditation or recitation of the *Gayatri Mantra*.

* **Technique** Raise the hands to the height of the face. With the elbows pointing down, turn the palms toward the face. Keep the hands about shoulder width apart.

* **Application** Sit in a quiet place, facing east (preferably at sunrise). Relax the shoulders and raise the hands into position. Feel your hands become soft and warm. Visualize the light of the rising sun shining upon your body. Imagine that this warm light radiates through your palms into your face, filling your body with light from head to toe.

* **Benefits** Activates the body's self-healing capacity, strengthens the immune system, assists the healing of serious diseases such as cancer, evokes feelings of devotion and surrender.

Mahashirsha Mudra

महाशीर्षमुद्रा

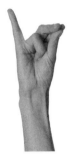

English "great head"

Devanagari महाशीर्षमुद्रा

Transliteration Mahāśīrṣamudrā

◈ **Description** *Mahashirsha Mudra* is a single-hand gesture (*asamyukta hasta*) common to the yoga tradition. It is used to relieve tension and balance the body's various energies.

◈ **Technique** Join the tips of the index and middle fingers together with the thumb. Curl the ring finger down into the palm of the hand and extend the little finger.

◈ **Application** In a comfortable seated position, form the mudra with each hand, resting the hands in the lap, palms up. Place the tip of the tongue on the upper palate. Relax the eyes, lips, and throat. Breathe naturally, resting your attention lightly on the navel. Hold for 5 to 20 minutes.

◈ **Benefits** Relieves headaches, reduces tension in the eyes, breaks up congestion in the frontal sinuses, improves mental clarity.

NOTE For chronic headaches, practice three shorter sessions of 5 to 10 minutes throughout the day. You may also practice the mudra lying down, followed by a brisk walk.

MAHATRIKA MUDRA

महात्रिकमुद्रा

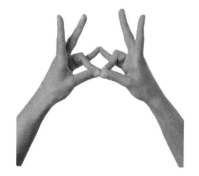

English "great sacrum," "triangular," or "trinity"

Devanagari महात्रिकमुद्रा

Transliteration Mahātrikamudrā

  ❋ **Description** *Mahatrika Mudra* is a joint-hand gesture (*samyukta hasta*) used in the yoga tradition to activate the healing energy of the pelvic area. This gesture works with the relationship between the Elements of Water (little finger), Fire (thumb), and Earth (ring finger) to harmonize the related organ systems inside the body.

  ❋ **Technique** With the palms of both hands facing each other, join the tips of the ring fingers. Then, touch the tips of the thumbs and little fingers, forming two rings. When performed correctly, the mudra resembles the bony structure of the human pelvis (as if looking from above down into the pelvic bowl).

  ❋ **Application** In a comfortable seated position, hold the mudra in front of the pubic bone. Soften the pelvic floor, belly, and chest. Place the tip of the tongue lightly against the upper palate. Breathe naturally. Hold for 5 to 45 minutes. To increase the healing potential of this mudra, practice 2 to 3 shorter sessions per day.

  ❋ **Benefits** Reduces menstrual cramping, regulates menstrual cycle, relieves pelvic congestion and constipation, benefits the prostate and bladder, aids the healing of hemorrhoids, assists the release of past emotions related to unconscious sex or sexual abuse.

Makara Mudra I

मकरमुद्रा

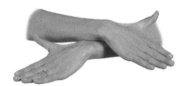

English "crocodile"

Devanagari मकरमुद्रा

Transliteration Makaramudrā

⁕ **Description** *Makara Mudra I* is a joint-hand dance gesture (*samyukta hasta*) noted in the *Natya Shastra* and in the *Abhinaya Darpana*. The patron deity associated with it is *Mahendra*.[27]

⁕ **Technique** Palms facing downward, form *Ardhachandra Mudra* (p.48) with each hand and cross the wrists. Thumbs move in circular motion.

⁕ **Application** Used to denote the sea, flow of the river, prosperity, solidarity, platform, crocodile, shark, fish, lion, tiger, elephant, and deer.

मकरमुद्रा

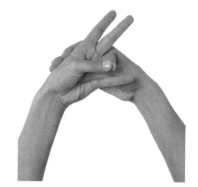

English "crocodile" or "mythical sea creature"

Devanagari मकरमुद्रा

Transliteration Makaramudrā

⁕ **Description** *Makara Mudra II* is a joint-hand gesture (*samyukta hasta*) used in the yoga tradition to symbolize water and fertility, and as a way to access the hidden mystical power of the Water Element. In Hindu and Buddhist art and architecture, *Makara* is considered an auspicious symbol, which represents the confluence of the *Ganga* and *Varuna* rivers, the sign of Capricorn, and the emblem of *Kama*, the god of love. This mythological sea creature can be seen carved in the cross bars of temples and monuments such as the *Great Stupa at Sanchi.*[28]

⁕ **Technique** Join the tips of the thumb and ring finger of your left hand. Insert the right thumb into the web between the left little and ring fingers, resting the tip of the right thumb at the base of the left thumb. Hold the right palm against the back of your left hand.

⁕ **Application** In a comfortable seated position, hold the mudra in front of the navel. Soften the belly and adjust your breathing to be slow, smooth, and deep. Feel the navel rising with the inhalation and descending with the exhalation. Expand your attention to include your lower back. Feel your kidneys and adrenal glands. Visualize an ocean of deep blue water there. Imagine that the power of this water is nourishing your kidneys and your entire body. Hold for 5 to 45 minutes.

⁕ **Benefits** Improves memory, strengthens the kidneys, benefits the sexual organs, helps to relieve low back pain, nourishes the hair, restores energy reserves.

MANDALA MUDRA

मण्डलमुद्रा

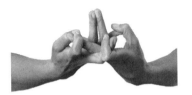

English "circular," "complete orbit," "essential ground," or "circling the center"

Devanagari मण्डलमुद्रा

Transliteration Maṇḍalamudrā

Additional Name *Tantra Linga*

FRONT VIEW

❋ **Description** *Mandala Mudra* is a joint-hand gesture (*samyukta hasta*) common to the traditions of Indian Tantrism and *Vajrayana* Buddhism. It is a ritual gesture representing a complete picture of the universe with Mount Meru[29] in the center and the four directions all around. It also symbolizes the ground of all creation, and the manifestation of specific deities such as *Tara* (in the context of Tantric Buddhism).

❋ **Technique** With the palms facing up, cross the little fingers and hold them down firmly with the thumbs. Cross the middle fingers and extend them straight. Hook the middle fingers with the index and root them down toward the palm. Press the backs of the ring fingers together, pointing them straight up.

❋ **Application** In a comfortable seated position, hold the mudra in front of the solar plexus (below the sternum). Lengthen the spine and relax the shoulders. Tuck the chin toward the chest gently, lengthening the back of the neck. Breathe naturally. Looking down, lightly focus your gaze on the tips of the extended ring fingers. You are looking at a symbolic model of the whole universe. Feeling the sincere wish for the welfare of all beings, offer this mandala to the limitless compassion

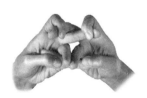

TOP VIEW

residing in the center of your own heart—your own Original Nature. Rest in this contemplation for 5 to 45 minutes.

☀ **Benefits** Awakens supreme devotion and enlightened attitude, improves concentration, evokes insight into the transitory nature of all things, serves as a physical expression of our own Original Nature.

MANIPURA CHAKRA MUDRA

मणिपूरचक्रमुद्रा

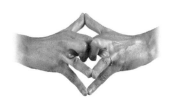

English "filled with jewels"

Devanagari मणिपूरचक्रमुद्रा

Transliteration Maṇipūracakramudrā

* **Description** *Manipura Chakra Mudra* is a complex joint-hand gesture (*samyukta hasta*) found in the yoga tradition and in esoteric Japanese martial arts. It relates to the *Manipura Chakra* (the navel center) in Indian Tantrism.

* **Technique** With both palms facing down, extend the index finger of the left hand and lift the left middle finger a little. Place the right index on top of the left index, slide it under the right middle finger, and rest the tip on top of the left ring finger. Bend the left middle finger down and curl the right middle finger over the top of the left index, so the two middle fingers sit side by side, and the tip of the left index finger sits on top of the right ring finger.

* **Application** In a comfortable seated position, hold the mudra in front of the solar plexus. Imagine a glowing ball of golden-red light in your belly. Rest in stillness and breathe naturally. Hold for 5 to 30 minutes.

* **Benefits** Strengthens digestion, improves the health of the liver, gall bladder, spleen, stomach, pancreas, and small and large intestine, bolsters willpower, improves martial ability, increases personal magnetism.

मन्मथमुद्रा

English "god of love and passion" or "churner of hearts"

Devanagari मन्मथमुद्रा

Transliteration Manmathamudrā

Additional names *Kamadeva, Makaradhwaja, Manasija, Pushpabana, Madana*

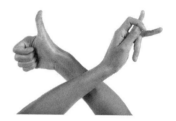

❋ **Description** *Manmatha Mudra* is a joint-hand gesture (*samyukta hasta*) used by performing artists. It is found in the traditional set of sixteen *Deva Hastas*, denoting Hindu gods and goddesses as described in the *Abhinaya Darpana*. It indicates the form and character of the Hindu deity *Manmatha*. He is most commonly depicted holding a bow and arrow, as he is known for shooting the five flower-arrows of sensual desire, intoxicating his "victims" with uncontrollable love and passion.

❋ **Technique** Assume *Shikhara Mudra* (p.225) with your left hand and *Katakamukha Mudra III* (p.122) with your right hand. Hold the hands either across from each other, or with the left arm stretched obliquely to your left at shoulder height, and the right hand held by the right shoulder as if shooting an arrow.

❋ **Application** Used to indicate *Manmatha*, the Hindu god of love and passion.

NOTE There are several combinations of mudras used to express the various traits and emblems of *Manmatha Deva*. The one indicated here appears to be the most common.

MATANGI MUDRA
मातङ्गिमुद्रा

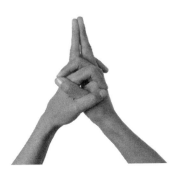

English "*devi* of inner harmony" or "guardian of outsiders and misfits"

Devanagari मातङ्गिमुद्रा

Transliteration Mātaṅgimudrā

❁ **Description** *Matangi Mudra* is a joint-hand gesture (*samyukta hasta*) used in yoga and Indian Tantrism to evoke the power of *Devi Matangi*, one of the ten *Mahavidyas*, or manifestations of the Divine Mother. *Matangi* is said to be the guardian of misfits and outsiders, who frowns upon the orthodox system of castes and the hypocrisy of society's high culture.

❁ **Technique** Interlace the fingers of both hands. Extend the middle fingers straight up, with the pads of the two fingers touching. Form two rings with the index fingers and thumbs of both hands.

❁ **Application** In a comfortable seated position, hold the mudra in front of the solar plexus. Lengthen the spine, and relax the chest and belly. Adjust your breathing to be slow, smooth, and deep. Use your inner power of discrimination to see through all the trappings of chasing status and position. In the silence of your own heart, release all contrivance and return to your original innocence. Hold for 5 to 45 minutes.

❁ **Benefits** Facilitates diaphragmatic breathing, benefits the abdomen and abdominal organs of digestion, assimilation, and elimination, activates the power of spirit, improves discernment and self-honesty, improves the voice and ability to communicate inner feelings.

Matri Mudra

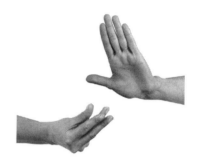

मातृमुद्रा

English "mother"

Devanagari मातृमुद्रा

Transliteration Mātṛmudrā

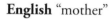

- **Description** *Matri Mudra* is a joint-hand gesture (*samyukta hasta*) used by performing artists. It is found in the traditional set of the eleven relationships (*Bandava Hastas*) as described in the *Abhinaya Darpana*. It indicates mother.

- **Technique** Assume *Ardhachandra Mudra* (p.48) with your left hand and *Samdamsha Mudra* (p.206) with your right hand. The left hand can be placed on the stomach indicating *Stri* (woman), which can mean daughter or mother, depending on the context.

- **Application** This gesture denotes mother or daughter.

MATSYA MUDRA I

मत्स्यमुद्रा

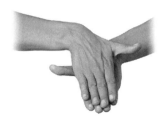

English "fish"

Devanagari मत्स्यमुद्रा

Transliteration Matsyamudrā

⁂ **Description** *Matsya Mudra I* is the seventeenth hand gesture of the twenty-four joint-hand mudras (*samyukta hastas*) as described in the *Abhinaya Darpana.*

⁂ **Technique** Place the right palm over the back your left hand, both palms facing downward. Keep all fingers collected, while extending the thumbs to the sides.

⁂ **Application** This mudra denotes a fish. Move your thumbs in circles to create a wave-like motion to express the movement of swimming. *Matsya* is known in the Hindu tradition as the first incarnation ("*avatara*") of *Vishnu.*

NOTE This mudra resembles *Makara Mudra.*

मत्स्यमुद्रा

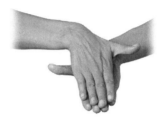

English "fish"

Devanagari मत्स्यमुद्रा

Transliteration Matsyamudrā

❋ **Description** *Matsya Mudra II* is a joint-hand gesture (*samyukta hasta*) common to the yoga tradition where it symbolizes one of the auspicious forms *Vishnu* assumed to benefit humanity. It is found in the *Yoga Tattva Mudra Vijnana* form, and is one of the traditional thirty-two *Gayatri Mudra*s, specifically the eighteenth gesture in the sub-set of twenty-four mudras practiced before meditation or recitation of the *Gayatri Mantra*.

❋ **Technique** Place your right palm over the back of your left hand, both palms facing downward. Keep all fingers collected, while extending the thumbs to the sides.

❋ **Application** In a comfortable seated position, lengthen the spine and relax the chest, shoulders, and belly. Hold the mudra in front of the abdomen and breathe naturally. Hold for 5 to 30 minutes.

❋ **Benefits** Activates the body's self-healing potential, increases suppleness, improves concentration, generates feelings of devotion and compassion.

Mayura Mudra I

मयूरमुद्रा

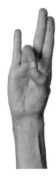

English "peacock"

Devanagari मयूरमुद्रा

Transliteration Mayūramudrā

Additional Name *Vajrapataka*

✳ **Description** *Mayura Mudra I* is the fifth hand gesture of the twenty-eight single-hand mudras (*asamyukta hastas*) as described in the *Abhinaya Darpana*. The name *Vajrapataka Mudra* is common to the Hindu tradition and it denotes the *vajra* (thunderbolt, weapon of *Indra*).

✳ **Technique** Raise the hand, palm facing forward, fingers collected and extended upward. Maintain active fingers and a flat palm. Join the tips of the ring finger and the thumb.

✳ **Application** Primarily used by performing artists to create context and express emotional states or specific actions. *Viniyoga*: *Mayurasyam* ("peacock beak"); *Latayancha* ("creeper vine"); *Shakuna* ("bird of omen"); *Vamana* ("vomiting"); *Alakashya-apanayana* ("stroking the hair" or "decorating the forehead"); *Lalata-tilakam-shucha* ("placing *tilak*[30] on the forehead"); *Nadi-udakasya-niksheypam* ("sprinkling holy water over the head"); *Shastra-vada* ("discussing the *shastras*"); *Prasidhaka* ("renown").

मयूरमुद्रा

English "peacock"

Devanagari मयूरमुद्रा

Transliteration Mayūramudrā

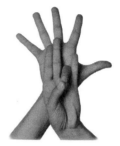

* **Description** This variation of *Mayura Mudra* is a joint-hand gesture (*samyukta hasta*) used in the dance tradition to depict a peacock.

* **Technique** Raise your left hand by your chest; palm faces outward, fingers spread wide to resemble the open tail of a peacock. Place your right hand in front of your left, forming *Mayura Mudra I* or *Kapittha Mudra* (p.106).

* **Application** Used in the dance tradition to depict a peacock, an iconographic symbol of immortality and love in Indian tradition.

MESHAYUDHA MUDRA
मेषयुधमुद्रा

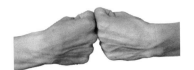

English "mighty deed" or "sheep fighting"

Devanagari मेषयुधमुद्रा

Transliteration Meṣayudhamudrā

* **Description** *Meshayudha Mudra* is a joint-hand gesture (*samyukta hasta*) noted in the *Abhinaya Chandrika*.

* **Technique** Form *Mushti Mudra* (p.163) with each hand, pressing the knuckles of the two hands together.

* **Application** Used in the dance tradition to illustrate struggle, war, forceful actions, or fighting between two entities.

MILITA ARDHAPATAKA MUDRA
मिलितार्धपताकमुद्रा

English "joint half-flag"

Devanagari मिलितार्धपताकमुद्रा

Transliteration Militārdhapatākamudrā

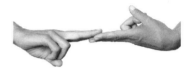

❋ **Description** *Milita Ardhapataka Mudra* is a joint-hand gesture (*samyukta hasta*) mentioned in the *Odissi Dance Pathfinder Vol. II.*

❋ **Technique** Form *Ardhapataka Mudra* (p.50) with each hand, joining the tips of the index and middle fingers of the two hands. Hold one hand facing upward, the other downward.

❋ **Application** This mudra is used in a common *chari* (transitional phrase) known as *Kutana*. Alternate the hands from downward facing to upward facing while dancing.

Mrigashirsha Mudra

मृगशीर्षमुद्रा

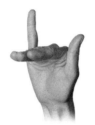

English "deer head"

Devanagari मृगशीर्षमुद्रा

Transliteration Mṛgaśīrṣamudrā

Additional Name *Chandra-mriga*

* **Description** *Mrigashirsha Mudra* is the seventeenth hand gesture of the twenty-eight single-hand mudras (*asamyukta hastas*) as described in the *Abhinaya Darpana*. It is also noted in the *Natya Shastra*. According to mythology, this mudra originated from *Gauri*,[31] when she drew three lines on her forehead while practicing *tapas*[32] to attract *Shiva's* attention. The associated sage is *Markandeya*, race is *Rishi*, color is white, and patron deity is *Maheshvara*.

* **Technique** With hand raised, extend the little finger and thumb upward, with the remaining fingers bent 90 degrees to the palm.

* **Application** Primarily used by performing artists to create context and express emotional states or specific actions. *Viniyoga*: *Strinam-artha* ("women's reproductive organs"); *Kapoola* ("cheek"); *Maryadayoh* ("traditional manners" or "limit"); *Bhityam* ("fear"); *Vivadam* ("argument"); *Nepathya* ("costume and make-up"); *Ahwane* ("calling" or "residence"); *Tripundraka* (drawing three lines on forehead); *Mriga-mukha* ("deer face"); *Rangavalayam* ("decorating the ground with patterns"); *Pada-samvahanam* ("foot massage"); *Sarvasammelane Karya* ("gathering all"); *Mandire* ("house"); *Chatra-dharana* ("holding an umbrella"); *Sopane* ("stairs"); *Padvinyasa* ("movement of the feet"); *Priya-ahvana* ("inviting the beloved"); *Samchara* ("roaming"). Additional usages denote: wall, deliberation, opportunity, screen, order, and body.

मृत्संजीवनीमुद्रा

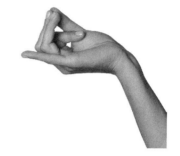

English "lifesaving gesture"

Devanagari मृत्संजीवनीमुद्रा

Transliteration Mṛtsaṁjīvanīmudrā

Additional Name *Apana Vayu*

❋ **Description** *Mritsamjivani Mudra* is a single-hand gesture (*asamyukta hasta*) common to the *Yoga Tattva Mudra Vijnana* form. It is used in the yoga tradition to benefit the heart, and as first aid for acute heart problems.

❋ **Technique** Place the index finger against the base of the thumb. Lightly join the tips of the middle and ring fingers with the tip of the thumb. Extend the little finger.

❋ **Application** In a comfortable seated position, form the mudra with each hand and rest the hands lightly on the thighs. Adjust your breathing to become slow and silent. Feel the chest and abdomen become soft and spacious. Hold for 5 to 45 minutes.

❋ **Benefits** Strengthens the heart and pericardium, regulates blood pressure, improves circulation and the health of arteries and veins, awakens the spirit of self-care and self-reflection, serves as a reminder to slow down and nurture body, mind, and spirit.

NOTE To aid recovery of chronic heart disease, and generally to increase the self-healing effects of this mudra, practice 2 to 3 sessions per day for a period of 100 days. In case of acute heart trouble, *Mritsamjivani Mudra* may be used as temporary support while awaiting help from an authorized medical professional.

MUDGARA MUDRA

मुद्गरमुद्रा

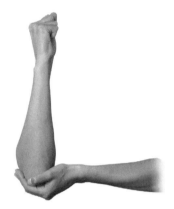

English "hammer-like weapon" or "club of Hanuman"

Devanagari मुद्गरमुद्रा

Transliteration Mudgaramudrā

Additional Name *Mugdharam*

❋ **Description** *Mudgara Mudra* is a joint-hand gesture (*samyukta hasta*) common to the yoga tradition. It is found in the *Yoga Tattva Mudra Vijnana* form, and is one of the traditional thirty-two *Gayatri Mudras*, specifically the twenty-third gesture in the sub-set of twenty-four mudras practiced before meditation or recitation of the *Gayatri Mantra*.

❋ **Technique** Place the left palm under the right side of the chest. Form a fist with the right hand, resting the right elbow in the palm of the left hand. Keep the right forearm vertical.

❋ **Application** In a comfortable seated position, relax the shoulders and breathe naturally. Imagine you are holding a weapon that defeats all your "inner demons" and reveals your true grace and talent. Hold for 5 to 30 minutes.

❋ **Benefits** Increases courage, virtue, and loyalty, stimulates the immune system, activates the body's self-healing power, and, according to the yoga tradition, facilitates the healing of major diseases such as cancer.

MUKULA MUDRA

मुकुलमुद्रा

English "bud" or "closed"

Devanagari मुकुलमुद्रा

Transliteration Mukulamudrā

Additional Name *Sukri*

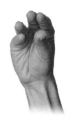

IMAGE I

❋ **Description** *Mukula Mudra* is the twenty-sixth hand gesture of the twenty-eight single-hand mudras (*asamyukta hastas*) as described in the *Abhinaya Darpana*. It is also noted in the *Natya Shastra*. According to mythology, this mudra originated from the monkey-god *Hanuman* when he attempted to seize the sun from the sky, mistaking it for a ripe *bimba* fruit. The associated sage is *Visakhila*, race is *Sankirna*, color is white, and patron deity is *Chandra*, the moon.

❋ **Technique** Variation 1: Join the tips of all five fingers (Image I). Variation 2: Bring the tips of all the fingers close together without touching (Image II)

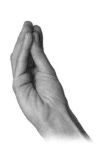

IMAGE II

❋ **Application** Primarily used by performing artists to create context and express emotional states or specific actions. *Viniyoga*: *Kumudha* ("water-lily"); *Bhoojana* ("eating"); *Pancha-bhana* ("five flower arrows of the god of love"); *Mudra-adi-dharana* ("holding a seal"); *Nabhi* ("navel"); *Kadli-pushpa* ("plantain flower"). Additional usages denote: charity, prayer, humbleness, lotus bud, self, life, passion, kissing children, folding an umbrella, and accepting fruit.

MULADHARA MUDRA

मूलाधारमुद्रा

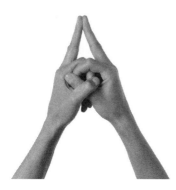

English "root support"

Devanagari मूलाधारमुद्रा

Transliteration Mūlādhāramudrā

* **Description** *Muladhara Mudra* is a lesser-known joint-hand mudra (*samyukta hasta*) used in Tantric Yoga and esoteric Japanese martial arts. It is related to the *Muladhara Chakra* (root center, the energy center at the base of the spine) in the Indian Tantric tradition.

* **Technique** Turn both palms to face upward. Interlace the little and ring fingers of both hands, so that the fingers fold inward toward the palms. Extend the middle fingers, joining them at the tips. Join the tips of the index fingers and thumbs of both hands, forming two interlocking rings.

* **Application** In a comfortable seated position, hold the mudra in the lap, in front of the pubic bone. Relax the belly and breathe naturally. Bring your attention to the perineum, located between the genitals and anus. Begin to contract and release the musculature of the pelvic floor and anus at about one contraction per second. Rest when you feel tired. Practice 2 to 3 sessions per day, building the duration of the sessions, as you get stronger.

* **Benefits** Improves elimination of waste, tones the muscles and organs of the pelvis, heals incontinence and hemorrhoids, increases sexual hormone production, increases fertility, creates stability and centeredness.

NOTE For women, the ideal point of contraction is located more deeply inside the vaginal canal, near the cervix. To develop sensitivity, and confirm you are contracting the correct area, gently insert one finger into the vagina as far as it will go. Then, contract the vaginal muscles in and upward against your finger multiple times.

मुष्टिमुद्रा

English "fist"

Devanagari मुष्टिमुद्रा

Transliteration Muṣṭimudrā

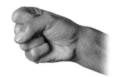

❋ **Description** *Mushti Mudra I* is the ninth hand gesture of the twenty-eight single-hand mudras (*asamyukta hastas*) as described in the *Abhinaya Darpana*. It is also noted in the *Natya Shastra*. According to mythology, this mudra originated from *Vishnu*, who used *Mushti Mudra* while fighting with the demon *Madhu*. The associated sage is *Indra*, race is *Shudra*, color is indigo, and patron deity is *Chandra*, the Moon.

❋ **Technique** Form a fist with the thumb on the outside of the other fingers.

❋ **Application** *Viniyoga*: *Sthiram* ("steadiness"); *Kachagraha* ("grasping one's hair"); *Dardhya* ("courage" or "firmness"); *Vasthvadeenamcha-dharana* ("holding things"); *Malianam-yudhabava* ("wrestling"). Additional usages denote: grasping, without bias, fruit, agreement, saying "very well," sacrificial offering, greeting common people, strong hold, holding a bell, running, lightness, holding a shield, fisticuffs, and grasping a spear.

Mushti Mudra II

मुष्टिमुद्रा

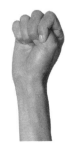

English "fist"

Devanagari मुष्टिमुद्रा

Transliteration Muṣṭimudrā

❋ **Description** *Mushti Mudra II* is a single-hand gesture (*asamyukta hasta*) common to the yoga tradition where it is used to consolidate *prana* (life force) in the *kanda* (lower belly).[33]

❋ **Technique** Touch the tip of the thumb to the base of the ring finger. Close the remaining fingers around the thumb to form a fist.

❋ **Application** In a comfortable seated position, form the mudra with each hand, resting the hands against the lower belly. Lightly contract the anus, while relaxing the belly and breathing naturally. Rest your attention on the space inside the body above the anus and below the navel. Hold for 5 to 45 minutes.

❋ **Benefits** Reduces anxiety and nervousness, strengthens digestion and assimilation, eliminates nightmares, calms the mind, imparts a sense of centeredness within the body, reduces fatigue and increases overall vitality.

Note For improved results, hold this mudra with each hand three times a day for 5 to 15 minutes. May be practiced while seated, standing, walking, or reclining.

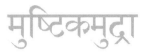
मुष्टिकमुद्रा

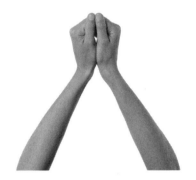

English "joined fist offering"

Devanagari मुष्टिकमुद्रा

Transliteration Muṣṭikamudrā

※ **Description** *Mushtika Mudra* is a joint-hand gesture (*samyukta hasta*) common to the yoga tradition. It is found in the *Yoga Tattva Mudra Vijnana* form, and is one of the traditional thirty-two *Gayatri Mudras*, specifically the seventeenth gesture in the sub-set of twenty-four mudras practiced before meditation or recitation of the *Gayatri Mantra*.

※ **Technique** Curl the fingers of each hand in toward the palm, making a fist. Join the hand together with the thumbs side by side.

※ **Application** In a comfortable seated position, hold the mudra lightly against your chest. Relax the shoulders, throat, and neck. Breathe naturally. Imagine there is a precious jewel of incalculable value inside your hands. This represents who you truly are, your unique gifts and talents. With sincerity in your heart, make an offering of the jewel internally as a commitment to live your life for the welfare of all beings. Do this repeatedly until tears of compassion flow from your eyes.

※ **Benefits** Weakens ego-grasping and self-defeating habits, awakens enlightened attitude and the heart of compassion, reduces anxiety and self-doubt, calms the spirit, clears the mind, benefits the heart and vascular system.

NOTE As you make the offering internally, you may also whisper the incantation, "I dedicate my thoughts, words, and actions to the welfare of all beings."

MUSHTIMRIGA MUDRA
मुष्टिमृगमुद्रा

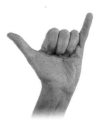

English "fist deer"

Devanagari मुष्टिमृगमुद्रा

Transliteration Muṣṭimṛgamudrā

✳ **Description** *Mushtimriga Mudra* is a single-hand gesture (*asamyukta hasta*) common to the dance tradition. In the *Abhinaya Darpana,* it is noted as one of the gestures that indicate "wild animals."

✳ **Technique** Fold the ring, middle, and index fingers into the palm, and extend the thumb and little finger outward and upward.

✳ **Application** Used in the dance tradition to denote a black antelope.

NAGABANDHA MUDRA

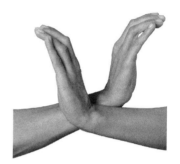

नागबन्धमुद्रा

English "serpent tie"

Devanagari नागबन्धमुद्रा

Transliteration Nāgabandhamudrā

❋ **Description** *Nagabandha Mudra* is the twenty-first hand gesture of the twenty-four joint-hand mudras (*samyukta hastas*) as described in the *Abhinaya Darpana.*

❋ **Technique** Cross your hands at the wrists with the two hands facing opposite each other. Curve your fingers to form the hood of a snake, as in *Sarpashirsha Mudra* (p.213).

❋ **Application** Primarily used by performing artists to create context and express emotional states or specific actions. *Viniyoga*: *Bhujanga-dampatibhava* ("pair of snakes"); *Nikunjanam Darshana* ("bowers"); *Atharvanasya Mantreshu* ("*Atharva-Veda* chants").

Nalini Padmakosha Mudra
नालिनीपद्मकोशमुद्रा

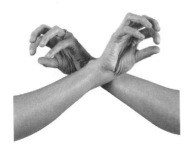

English "fragrant lotus buds"

Devanagari नालिनीपद्मकोशमुद्रा

Transliteration Nālinīpadmakośamudrā

⚜ **Description** *Nalini Padmakosha Mudra* is a joint-hand gesture (*samyukta hasta*) common to the dance tradition. It is noted in the *Abhinaya Darpana*. The patron deity associated with this mudra is *Shesha*.[34]

⚜ **Technique** Cross the wrists and turn your palms outward. Separate your fingers and thumb and gently curl them inward toward the hollowed palms without touching the tips. Keep your hands in front of your torso, about 6 inches away from your body.

⚜ **Application** Used to denote entwined snakes, flower buds, a cluster of flowers, making equal distributions, the number ten, and a type of bird.

NANANDRI MUDRA

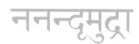

ननन्दृमुद्रा

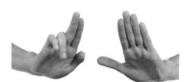

English "sister-in-law"

Devanagari ननन्दृमुद्रा

Transliteration Nanandṛmudrā

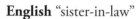

❋ **Description** *Nanandri Mudra* is a joint-hand gesture (*samyukta hasta*) used by performing artists. It is found in the traditional set of the eleven relationships (*Bandava Hastas*) as described in the *Abhinaya Darpana*. It indicates sister-in-law.

❋ **Technique** Form *Mrigashirsha Mudra* (p.158) with your left hand and place it on your stomach (this is called the *stri* "feminine" hand). Form *Kartarimukha Mudra* (p.115) or *Shikhara Mudra* (p.225) with your right hand.

❋ **Application** This gesture denotes sister-in-law.

NETRA MUDRA I
नेत्रमुद्रा

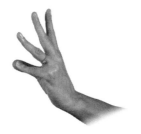

English "eye"

Devanagari नेत्रमुद्रा

Transliteration Netramudrā

❋ **Description** *Netra Mudra I* is a single-hand gesture (*asamyukta hasta*) common to Hindu and Buddhist traditions. It is a ritual gesture used to represent an eye, usually symbolizing the power of a particular deity to see through confusion and ignorance.

❋ **Technique** Join the tips of the thumb and little finger. Extend the remaining fingers upward.

❋ **Application** Hold the mudra in front of the eye, so that you can see through the hole.

NOTE This mudra is primarily used in the context of ritual and is not described as having particular healing benefits for the individual.

नेत्रमुद्रा

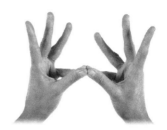

English "eye"

Devanagari नेत्रमुद्रा

Transliteration Netramudrā

* **Description** *Netra Mudra II* is the joint-hand version (*samyukta hasta*) of *Netra Mudra I*. It is a ritual gesture used in Hindu and Buddhist traditions during *puja* or *yajna* to depict the eyes of a deity such as *Kali* or *Tara*.

* **Technique** Join the tips of the thumbs and little fingers of each hand. Extend the remaining fingers upward. Bring the two hands together, touching the tips of the little fingers and thumbs in the center.

* **Application** Raise the mudra in front of the eyes.

NOTE This mudra is primarily used in the context of ritual and is not described as having particular healing benefits for the individual.

NIMBASALA MUDRA
निम्बसलमुद्रा

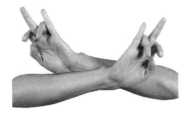

English "type of tree"

Devanagari निम्बसलमुद्रा

Transliteration Nimbasalamudrā

- ❋ **Description** *Nimbasala Mudra* is a joint-hand gesture (*samyukta hasta*) common to the dance tradition. In the *Abhinaya Darpana*, it is noted as one of the gestures that indicate "trees."

- ❋ **Technique** Assume *Shukatunda Mudra* (p.229) with both hands, and cross at the wrists. Palms face outward.

- ❋ **Application** Used in the dance tradition to denote the *Nimbasala* tree.

NOTE The word *nimba* by itself refers to the neem tree, which has many healing benefits and serves as a natural pesticide when planted near gardens.

NIRRITI MUDRA
निर्ऋतिमुद्रा

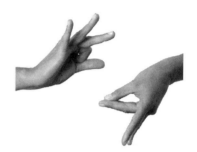

English "goddess of death and corruption"

Devanagari निर्ऋतिमुद्रा

Transliteration Nirṛtimudrā

Additional Name *Rakshasa*

❂ **Description** *Nirriti Mudra* is a joint-hand gesture (*samyukta hasta*) used by performing artists. It is found in the traditional set of sixteen *Deva Hastas*, denoting Hindu gods and goddesses as described in the *Abhinaya Darpana*. It indicates the form and character of the Hindu deity *Nirriti*.

❂ **Technique** Form *Khatva Mudra* (p.126) with your left hand and *Shakata Mudra* (p.214) with your right hand. Hold the left hand in front of your waist and the right hand in front of your chest.

❂ **Application** Used to indicate *Nirriti*, the goddess of death and corruption, and the guardian of the southwest direction. See Appendix C for a chart of the Guardians of the Eight Directions.

NOTE There are several combinations of mudras used to express the various traits and emblems of *Nirriti Devi*. The one indicated here appears to be the most common.

NIRVANA MUDRA
निर्वाणमुद्रा

English "liberation"

Devanagari निर्वाणमुद्रा

Transliteration Nirvāṇamudrā

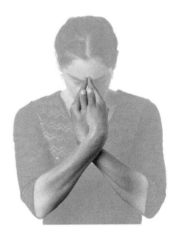

❋ **Description** *Nirvana Mudra* is an intricate joint-hand gesture (*samyukta hasta*) common to the yoga tradition. It is found in the *Yoga Tattva Mudra Vijnana* form, and is final gesture in the set of thirty-two traditional *Gayatri Mudras*, specifically the eighth mudra of the sub-set of eight gestures practiced after meditation or recitation of the *Gayatri Mantra*.

IMAGE I

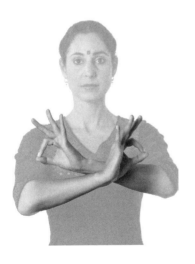

IMAGE II

❋ **Technique** Turn the left palm up and the right palm down. Move the right hand under the left, hooking the little, ring, and middle fingers of each hand. Move the left hand up in an arc, so that the palms of the two hands come together. Extend the index fingers, and join the tips together. Bring the thumbs side by side in the hollow space created by the index fingers. Gently rotate the mudra toward your body and upward, until the index fingers point straight up (Image I). Bow the head forward, touching the "third-eye center" to the tips of the index fingers. Hold for 1 to 2 minutes (longer if desired). Then, reverse the rotation, letting the mudra unwind itself. Form two *Jnana Mudras* (p.100), with the wrists crossed (Image II). Rotate the hands toward your body, bringing the hands palms up, little fingers touching. Conclude by bowing the head to the heels of the hands (Image III).

✺ **Application** Use *Nirvana Mudra* as a ritual gesture, symbolizing your commitment to realizing your own Original Nature in this very lifetime. Dedicate the benefit of your practice to the welfare of all beings. After a session of meditation or recitation of mantra, perform the movements of the mudra slowly and meticulously. Mentally gather all the benefits of your *sadhana* (personal practice) into the mudra and offer them to all beings.

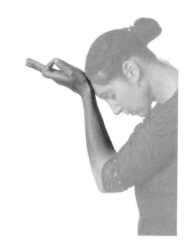

✺ **Benefits** Weakens ego grasping, reduces selfish desire for personal gain from spiritual practice, awakens the heart of compassion, serves as a ritual gesture to conclude any practice, as well as a simple way to "dedicate the merit."

IMAGE III

NOTE While performing *Nirvana Mudra*, you may also chant the prayer, *Lokah Samasthah Sukhino Bhavantu Om Shanti Shanti Shanti* ("May all beings everywhere be happy! Om Peace Peace and Eternal Peace"). This will add additional power and devotion to the application of the mudra.

Nishedha Mudra

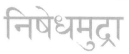
निषेधमुद्रा

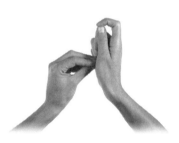

English "defense"

Devanagari निषेधमुद्रा

Transliteration Niṣedhamudrā

* **Description** *Nishedha Mudra* is a joint-hand gesture (*samyukta hasta*) noted in the *Abhinaya Darpana* and *Natya Shastra*. The patron deity associated with this gesture is *Tumburu*.[35]

* **Technique** Form *Mukula Mudra* (p.161) with your left hand and press the tips of your fingers against your right palm held in *Kapittha Mudra* (p.106).

* **Application** Indicates grasping, receiving, preserving, convention, truthfulness, and compression. Also used to worship the *Shivalinga* in *Anga Puja*.[36]

Nitamba Mudra

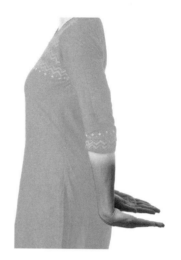

नितम्बमुद्रा

English "buttock"

Devanagari नितम्बमुद्रा

Transliteration Nitambamudrā

❋ **Description** *Nitamba Mudra* is a joint-hand dance gesture (*samyukta hasta*) noted in the *Natya Shastra* and *Abhinaya Darpana*. The patron deity associated is *Agastya*.[37]

❋ **Technique** Form *Pataka Mudra* (p.186) with each hand and place the hands behind the buttocks, palms up. Arms are extended downward. The dynamic version is to move your upward facing palms from shoulders to buttocks.

❋ **Application** In the dance tradition it is used to denote weariness, descent, astonishment, and ecstasy.

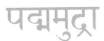 # PADMA MUDRA
पद्ममुद्रा

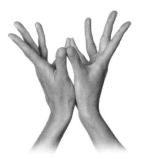

English "lotus flower"

Devanagari पद्ममुद्रा

Transliteration Padmamudrā

Additional names *Pankajam, Panka, Kamala Ghumana*

⁕ **Description** *Padma Mudra* is a joint-hand gesture (*samyukta hasta*) common to the Hindu, yoga, Tantric, and dance traditions. It is found in the *Yoga Tattva Mudra Vijnana* form and is one of the thirty-two traditional *Gayatri Mudras*, specifically the sixth gesture in the sub-set of eight mudras practiced after meditation or recitation of the *Gayatri Mantra*.

⁕ **Technique** Raise the hands in front of the heart center. Join the heels of the two palms while spreading the fingers upward to create a hollow space between the palms. The little fingers and thumbs may touch or stay slightly apart.

⁕ **Application (yoga)** In a comfortable seated position, hold the mudra in front of the heart. Soften the chest and belly, and adjust your breathing to be slow, smooth, and deep. With the eyelids half-drawn, gaze into the center of the lotus flower formed by the hands. Discard all contrivance and release all ambitions that are not in harmony with your "heart of hearts." Do this honestly within yourself. Resolve to make your life an offering for the benefit of all beings. Stay with this feeling for 5 to 45 minutes.

⁕ **Application (dance)** In dance, there is a dynamic application of this gesture executed by turning the wrists round and round each other continuously in a soft manner without losing contact. This is known as the offering of the "Heart Lotus." It is used to denote spiritual feelings of love, beauty, and grace.

❋ **Benefits** Weakens ego grasping, opens *Anahata Chakra*, settles the mind, benefits the heart and pericardium, balances the immune system, awakens the body's self-healing power, ignites spiritual devotion.

NOTE Although *Padma Mudra* is used in all forms of Classical Indian Dance, it is especially common to the North Indian dance, *Kathak*. The name *Kamala Ghumana* is derived from that tradition.

Padmakosha Mudra
पद्मकोशमुद्रा

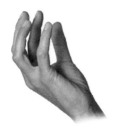

English "lotus bud"

Devanagari पद्मकोशमुद्रा

Transliteration Padmakośamudrā

❋ **Description** *Padmakosha Mudra* is the fifteenth hand gesture of the twenty-eight single-hand mudras (*asamyukta hastas*) as described in the *Abhinaya Darpana*. It is also noted in the *Natya Shastra*. According to mythology, it originated from *Narayana* when he was worshiping *Shiva* with lotus flowers to obtain his discus ("*sudarshana-chakra*"). The associated sage is *Padmadhara*, race is *Yaksha-Kinnara*, color is white, and patron deity is *Bhargava*.

❋ **Technique** Place your hand palm up with the fingers apart. Slightly bend all five fingers keeping the palm hollow.

❋ **Application** Primarily used by performing artists to create context and express emotional states or specific actions. *Viniyoga: Phale bilva-kapittha* ("various fruits"); *Strinam-cha-kutcha-kumbhayoh* ("round breasts of a woman"); *Avartake* ("circular movement"); *Kanduke* ("ball"); *Sthalyam* ("bowl"); *Bhojane* ("food"); *Pushpa-koraka* ("flower garland"); *Shakaraphala* ("mango"); *Pushpavarsha* ("showering flowers"); *Manjarika-adishu* ("cluster of flowers"); *Japakusuma* ("Hibiscus flower"); *Gantarupa Vidhanaka* ("bell shape" or "preparing a big bowl of food for elephants"); *Valmika* ("ant-hill"); *Kamala* ("lotus"); *Anda* ("egg"). Additional usages denote: elephant trunk, brilliance, vessel of gold or silver, coil of hair, moderation, charm, bending a bough, and coconut.

पल्लवमुद्रा

English "leaf"

Devanagari पल्लवमुद्रा

Transliteration Pallavamudrā

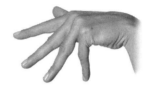

❋ **Description** *Pallava Mudra I* is noted in the *Abhinaya Darpana* and in the *Natya Shastra*. The *Abhinaya Darpana* describes it as a single-hand gesture (*asamyukta hasta*), while the *Natya Shastra* calls it a joint-hand gesture (*samyukta hasta*).

❋ **Technique** With the palm facing downward, bend the wrist and fan out the fingers. To form the joint-hand version, join the wrists and circle the hands around each other in a spiral-like motion. Move the hands up and down simulating leaves swirling in the wind.

❋ **Application** In the dance tradition, it is utilized in *Nritta* or "pure dance" to express delicate grace and beauty.

PALLAVA MUDRA II

पल्लवमुद्रा

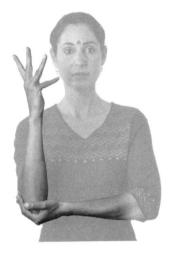

English "leaf swaying in the wind"

Devanagari पल्लवमुद्रा

Transliteration Pallavamudrā

❋ **Description** *Pallava Mudra II* is a single-hand gesture (*asamyukta hasta*) common to the yoga tradition. It is found in the *Yoga Tattva Mudra Vijnana* form, and is one of the traditional thirty-two *Gayatri Mudras*, specifically the last gesture in the sub-set of twenty-four mudras practiced before meditation or recitation of the *Gayatri Mantra*.

❋ **Technique** Raise the right hand in front of the right shoulder with the palm facing forward. Relax the hand and allow the fingers to separate and move slowly, as if each finger is a leaf swaying in the wind. Rest the right elbow in the left palm.

❋ **Application** In a comfortable seated position, hold the mudra for 5 to 30 minutes. Feel that you are a mighty tree. Your lower hand (left) digs down into the earth (roots), and your upper hand (right) stretches to the sky (leaves). Feel that you are breathing with your skin and lungs. As you breathe in, *prana* (energy) absorbs through your skin; as you breathe out, this energy consolidates in to your belly, deeply nourishing your body.

❋ **Benefits** Harmonizes all Five Elements, balances the immune system, activates the body's self-healing power, improves the suppleness of the joints, tendons, and ligaments.

पञ्चमुखमुद्रा

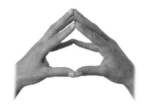

English "five faces"

Devanagari पञ्चमुखमुद्रा

Transliteration Pañcamukhamudrā

❋ **Description** *Panchamukha Mudra* is a joint-hand gesture (*samyukta hasta*) common to the yoga tradition. It is found in the *Yoga Tattva Mudra Vijnana* form, and is one of the traditional thirty-two *Gayatri Mudras*, specifically the eighth gesture in the sub-set of twenty-four mudras practiced before meditation or recitation of the *Gayatri Mantra*.

❋ **Technique** Join the tips of all of the fingers, hollowing the palms, as if holding a ball of light between the hands.

❋ **Application** In a comfortable seated position, hold the mudra in front of the solar plexus (below the navel). Relax the shoulders and chest, and breathe naturally. Hold for 5 to 45 minutes.

❋ **Benefits** Balances the left and right hemispheres of the brain (by affecting the corpus callosum, which acts as a bridge between the two hemispheres), improves concentration and memory retention, benefits the tendons, activates the body's self-healing power.

Parvati Mudra
पार्वतीमुद्रा

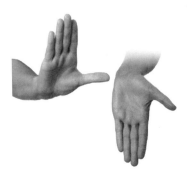

English "the divine mother"

Devanagari पार्वतीमुद्रा

Transliteration Pārvatīmudrā

* **Description** *Parvati Mudra* is a joint-hand gesture (*samyukta hasta*) used by performing artists. It is found in the traditional set of sixteen *Deva Hastas*, denoting Hindu gods and goddesses as described in the *Abhinaya Darpana*. It indicates the form and character of the Hindu deity *Parvati*.

* **Technique** Assume *Ardhachandra Mudra* (p.48) with each hand. Hold the right hand with fingers pointing upward and the left hand with fingers pointing downward; forming *Abhaya* (dispelling fear) and *Varada* (bestowing protection), respectively. Hold the hand gestures at waist height to the sides of your body about 6 inches in front of you. Assume the posture of *abhanga* (shifting your weight to one foot and slightly bending the torso).

* **Application** Used to indicate *Parvati*, the Hindu goddess known as the Divine Mother. She is the consort of *Shiva*.

NOTE There are several combinations of mudras used to express the various traits and emblems of *Parvati Devi*. The one indicated here appears to be the most common.

PASHA MUDRA

पाशमुद्रा

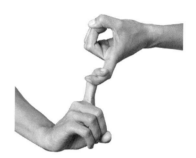

English "noose"

Devanagari पाशमुद्रा

Transliteration Pāśamudrā

❀ **Description** *Pasha Mudra* is the fifteenth hand gesture of the twenty-four joint-hand mudras (*samyukta hastas*) as described in the *Abhinaya Darpana*.

❀ **Technique** With the pads of the thumb, touch the nails of the middle, ring, and little fingers on each hand. Extend the index fingers and hook them together with one palm facing up, the other facing down.

❀ **Application** Primarily used by performing artists to create context and express emotional states or specific actions. *Viniyoga*: *Anyonya Kalaha* ("fighting" or "lovers' quarrel"); *Pasha* ("noose"); *Shrinkhalayam* ("chain").

Pataka Mudra

पताकमुद्रा

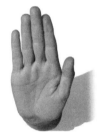

English "flag"

Devanagari पताकमुद्रा

Transliteration Patākamudrā

Additional Name *Dhvaja*

Description *Pataka Mudra* is the first hand gesture of the twenty-eight single-hand mudras (*asamyukta hastas*) as described in the *Abhinaya Darpana*. It is also noted in the *Natya Shastra* and *Abhinaya Chandrika* (as *Dhvaja*). This hand gesture is the most versatile of all dance mudras and has many meanings and usages. According to mythology, it originated when *Brahma* (the creator) went to *Parabrahma* (the supreme being) to salute him with his hand held like a flag, symbolizing victory. Since then, it has been called the "flag hand." The associated sage is *Shiva*, race is *Brahmana*, color is white, and patron deity is *Parabrahma*. It is very similar to *Abhaya Mudra*, used in Buddhism and in the yoga tradition.

Technique Hold your hand raised, palm facing forward, fingers extended upward. Bend your thumb slightly to touch the base of the index finger on the outside. Maintain active fingers and a flat palm.

Application Primarily used by performing artists to create context and express emotional states or specific actions. *Viniyoga*: *Natya-rambha* ("beginning of the dance or drama"); *Varivahay* ("rain clouds"); *Bhana* ("forest"); *Vasthu Nishaydhanay* ("forbidding or avoiding things"); *Kuchasithala* ("bosom"); *Nisayam* ("night"); *Nadyam* ("river"); *Amaramandala* ("heaven"); *Thuranga* ("horse"); *Kandhana* ("cutting" or "ignoring"); *Vayu* ("wind"); *Shayana* ("sleeping" or "reclining"); *Gamana-udyama* ("walking" or "embarking on a long journey"); *Pratapa* ("prowess"); *Prasada* ("blessing" or "graciousness"); *Chandrika* ("moonlight"); *Gana-atapa* ("intense radiance" or "scorching sunlight"); *Kavata-patanam* ("opening a door"); *Saptha-vibakthi-artham* ("mentioning the seven cases of grammar"); *Tharanga* ("wave"); *Veethipravaysha-*

bhava ("entering a street"); *Samathva* ("equality"); *Angaragaka* ("massaging" or "applying sandal paste"); *Athmartham* ("one's self"); *Shapatham* ("taking an oath"); *Thushneembhava-nidharshanam* ("silence" or "secret act"); *Talapathra* ("palm leaf"); *Kayday* ("shield"); *Dravyadi-sparshanam* ("touching things"); *Aashirvada Kriyayam* ("benediction"); *Nrupasreshtrasya Bhavana* ("a good king or emperor"); *Tatra-tatra-iti-vachanam* ("this and that"); *Sindhu* ("ocean wave"); *Sukrudikrama* ("to do good deeds"); *Sambhodhanam* ("addressing"—a person some distance away); *Purogaypee* ("to move forward"); *Khadgasya-rupadharana* ("holding a sword"); *Masa* ("month"); *Samvathsara* ("year"); *Varsadhina* ("rainy day"); *Sammarjana* ("sweeping the floor" or "to sprinkle water").

PHUPPHUSAMOCANA MUDRA

फुप्फुसमोचनमुद्रा

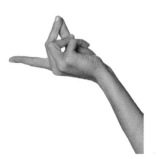

English "chest opening" or "lung freeing"

Devanagari फुप्फुसमोचनमुद्रा

Transliteration Phupphusamocanamudrā

❀ **Description** *Phupphusamocana Mudra* is a single-hand gesture (*asamyukta hasta*) used in the yoga tradition to ease depression, strengthen the lungs, and as first aid for acute lung problems such as asthma.

❀ **Technique** Touch the little finger to the base of the thumb, ring finger to the middle of the thumb, and middle finger to the tip of the thumb. Extend the index finger.

❀ **Application** Form the mudra with both hands. Raise your arms to your sides, shoulder height, and turn palms to face away from you. Lengthen the arms with gentle inner force, as if pushing two imaginary walls apart. Extend the index finger a little more. Relax the neck and shoulders, and breathe naturally (do not hold your breath). Feel your chest open and your back wide. Create more room to breathe. Hold as long as comfortable.

❀ **Benefits** Clears the airways, opens the chest, and improves the elasticity of the ribcage, facilitating ease of breathing, strengthens the immune system, specifically reducing susceptibility to lung-related complaints, helps the processing of grief and sadness, and helps lift the heaviness of depression.

NOTE In the beginning you may only be able to perform this exercise for a short time. With practice, you will learn to relax from within and let your breathing float your arms. This may be done seated or standing. Practice 3 to 5 sessions per day. Alternately, you may simply place the mudra in your lap and rest in stillness for 5 to 45 minutes.

CAUTION In the case of acute lung problems, mudras and other self-healing methods are best used in conjunction with professional medical care.

PITRI MUDRA

पितृमुद्रा

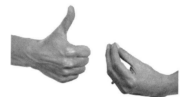

English "father"

Devanagari पितृमुद्रा

Transliteration Pitṛmudrā

* **Description** *Pitri Mudra* is a joint-hand gesture (*samyukta hasta*) used by performing artists. It is found in the traditional set of the eleven relationships (*Bandava Hastas*) as described in the *Abhinaya Darpana*. It indicates father or son-in-law.

* **Technique** Assume *Samdamsha Mudra* (p.206) with your left hand and *Shikhara Mudra* (p.225) with your right hand.

* **Application** This gesture denotes father or son-in-law, depending on the context of the performance.

PRABODHIKA MUDRA

प्रबोधिकमुद्रा

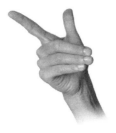

English "dawn"

Devanagari प्रबोधिकमुद्रा

Transliteration Prabodhikamudrā

* **Description** *Prabodhika Mudra* is a single-hand gesture (*asamyukta hasta*) noted in the *Abhinaya Chandrika*.

* **Technique** Extend the thumb and index fingers while bending the middle, ring, and little fingers loosely into the palm (without touching the palm).

* **Application** Used to convey the question, "Where are you?" usually in the context of yearning to unite with the beloved. It is similar in appearance to *Chandrakala Mudra*.

PRADEEPA MUDRA

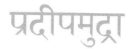

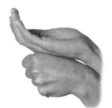

English "oil lamp"

Devanagari प्रदीपमुद्रा

Transliteration Pradīpamudrā

- **Description** *Pradeepa Mudra* is a joint-hand mudra (*samyukta hasta*) noted in the *Abhinaya Chandrika*.

- **Technique** Make a fist with your left hand. With the fingers curved upward, place the back of the right hand on top of the left fist.

- **Application** Used in the dance tradition to illustrate the Hindu ritual of offering light to the deities by circling an ignited oil lamp in front of the deity.[38]

Pralamba Mudra

प्रलम्बमुद्रा

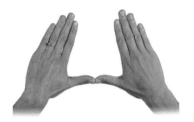

English "spread offerings" or "garland"

Devanagari प्रलम्बमुद्रा

Transliteration Pralambamudrā

✳ **Description** *Pralamba Mudra* is a joint-hand gesture (*samyukta hasta*) common to the yogic tradition. It is found in the *Yoga Tattva Mudra Vijnana* form, and is one of the traditional thirty-two *Gayatri Mudras*, specifically the sixteenth gesture in the sub-set of twenty-four mudras practiced before meditation or recitation of the *Gayatri Mantra*.

✳ **Technique** With the palms facing down, join the tips of the thumbs while keeping the other fingers collected.

✳ **Application** In a comfortable seated position, hold the mudra in front of the abdomen. Soften the hands and relax the shoulders. Open your heart to hear the wishes and prayers of all beings—our shared longing to be free and happy. Respond with sincere blessings that you feel emanate from your hands like a huge garland of pearls, encircling the entire universe. Hold the mudra and visualization for 5 to 30 minutes.

✳ **Benefits** Opens the heart, calms the spirit, awakens feelings of devotion and compassion, benefits the cardiovascular system by lowering blood pressure, reduces anxiety, weakens ego grasping.

प्राणमुद्रा

English "energy seal"

Devanagari प्राणमुद्रा

Transliteration Prāṇamudrā

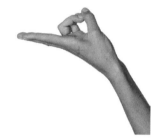

❋ **Description** *Prana Mudra* is a single-hand gesture (*asamyukta hasta*) common to numerous yoga traditions throughout Asia. It is part of the *Yoga Tattva Mudra Vijnana* form where it is used in recuperation from injury or illness, to increase energy reserves, and bolster the effects of other mudras. In the context of Buddhism and Asian martial arts, it is called "sword finger" or the "sword of wisdom," and is applied in a ritual manner to cut through ignorance and laziness, or in the context of martial and healing arts, to direct vital energy (*prana, qi, ki*).

❋ **Technique** Cover the tips of the ring and little fingers with the pad of the thumb. Extend the index and middle finger.

❋ **Application** In a comfortable seated position, form the mudra with each hand. With the extended fingers pointing forward, rest the hands against the sides of the abdomen. Lift the perineum and contract the anus firmly. Relax the chest and ribs, and adjust your breathing to be slow, smooth, and deep. Visualize a ball of golden-red light inside your abdomen. This ball of light is growing brighter with each breath. Hold in stillness for 5 to 45 minutes.

❋ **Benefits** Increases overall vitality and immunity, activates the body's self-healing potential, benefits the eyes, improves digestion, assimilation, and elimination, decreases the body's susceptibility to injury and disease, improves concentration, strengthens willpower and stamina.

NOTE *Prana Mudra* may be done anytime in any position, especially when feeling tired. It is especially useful during practice of standing yoga *asanas* (postures) where the arms are extended. In this case, the mudra increases the energetic effects of the pose or exercise. It may also be used as a healing tool to assist the body's innate capacity to repair itself. Hold the mudra about 6 inches away from the body with the "sword fingers" pointing toward the affected area. Breathe naturally and let go. Do not try to use your mind or will make energy move or cause a specific effect to occur. This same principle of non-action applies when using *Prana Mudra* for self-healing or helping others to heal.

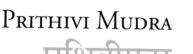

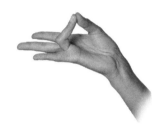

English "earth"

Devanagari पृथिवीमुद्रा

Transliteration Pṛthivīmudrā

* **Description** *Prithivi Mudra* is a joint-hand mudra (*samyukta hasta*) common to the yoga tradition. It is used in the *Yoga Tattva Mudra Vijnana* to affect the Earth Element for the purpose of improving digestion, and generally to strengthen the bodily constitution.

* **Technique** Lightly join the tips of the thumb and ring finger. The other fingers remain extended and relaxed.

* **Application** In a comfortable seated position, form the mudra with each hand. Rest the hands in the lap, palms facing up. Soften the ribs and belly, and adjust your breathing to be slow, smooth, and deep. Feel the belly rise with the inhalation and fall with the exhalation. Imagine a ball of golden-red light inside your abdomen growing brighter with each breath. Hold for 5 to 45 minutes.

* **Benefits** Strengthens digestion and assimilation, helps rebuild a thin and frail constitution, creates a sense of centeredness and grounding, benefits the skin, improves the disposition, helps one adjust to any kind of change or disruption to the normal schedule or routine; spiritually it establishes a sense of effortless joy.

NOTE *Prithivi Mudra* may be practiced while walking, standing, or lying down. Anytime you desire to feel more centered and grounded, such as before a presentation, exam, or long journey, you can employ this mudra discreetly.

PURNA JNANA MUDRA

पूर्णज्ञानमुद्रा

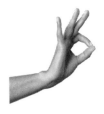

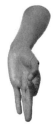

English "complete wisdom"

Devanagari पूर्णज्ञानमुद्रा

Transliteration Pūrṇajñānamudrā

Additional Name *Jnanam*

* **Description** *Purna Jnana Mudra* is a joint-hand mudra (*samyukta hasta*) used in the *Yoga Tattva Mudra Vijnana* form. It is one of the thirty-two *Gayatri Mudras*, specifically the second gesture in the sub-set of eight mudras practiced after meditation or recitation of the *Gayatri Mantra*.

* **Technique** Lightly join the tips of the thumbs and index fingers of both hands.

* **Application** In a comfortable seated position, form the mudra with each hand. Hold the right hand in front of the heart and rest the left hand on the knee, palm facing up. Relax the shoulders and chest, and breathe naturally. Release effort and any expectation for results. Simply relax into the texture of your own direct experience. Hold for 5 to 45 minutes.

* **Benefits** Opens the chest for ease of breathing, calms the heart and spirit, improves intelligence and ability to concentrate, expands feelings of compassion and care for self and others, serves as a gateway for discovering the innate wisdom arising in our own direct experience.

PUSHPA MUDRA

पुष्पमुद्रा

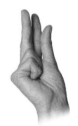

English "flower"

Devanagari पुष्पमुद्रा

Transliteration Puṣpamudrā

- **Description** *Pushpa Mudra* is a single-hand gesture (*asamyukta hasta*) noted in the *Abhinaya Chandrika*.

- **Technique** Bend the little and ring fingers and tuck them into the center of your palm. Extend the thumb, middle, and index fingers upward, forming a triangle between the fingertips.

- **Application** Used to denote a flower or flower offering in the dance tradition. It is also known in the Japanese Buddhist tradition as "the *bodhisattva* of flowers" and is used in specific rites and rituals to signify the offering of flowers.

PUSHPAPUTA MUDRA

पुष्पपुटमुद्रा

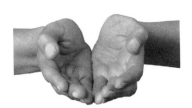

English "flower-vessel"

Devanagari पुष्पपुटमुद्रा

Transliteration Puṣpapuṭamudrā

Additional names *Pushpanjali, Kandajali, Vyapakanjalikam*

* **Description** *Pushpaputa Mudra* is the sixth hand gesture of the twenty-four joint-hand mudras (*samyukta hastas*) as described in the *Abhinaya Darpana*. It is also noted in the *Natya Shastra*. The patron deity associated with it is *Ksetrapala*.

* **Technique** With the palms facing upward, curve the hands and join the outer side of the little fingers, as if to create a basket-like shape in front of your heart center.

* **Application** Primarily used by performing artists to create context and express emotional states or specific actions. *Viniyoga*: *Nirajana-vidhau* ("offering light"); *Vari-phala-adigrahana* ("receiving fruit or water"); *Samdhyayam-arghya-dana* ("twilight offering to the sun"); *Mantra-pushpa* ("offering flowers while chanting"). It is generally used to offer and receive flowers, fruit, corn, rice, or water.

पुत्रमुद्रा

English "son"

Devanagari पुत्रमुद्रा

Transliteration Putramudrā

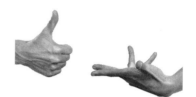

- **Description** *Putra Mudra* is a joint-hand gesture (*samyukta hasta*) used by performing artists. It is found in the traditional set of the eleven relationships (*Bandava Hastas*) as described in the *Abhinaya Darpana*. It indicates son. It replaces *Bhartri Mudra* ("husband") in some translations of the text.

- **Technique** Form *Alapadma Mudra* (p.41) with your left hand and *Shikhara Mudra* (p.225) with your right hand.

- **Application** This gesture denotes son.

RAHU MUDRA

राहुमुद्रा

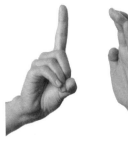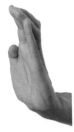

English "dragon's head"

Devanagari राहुमुद्रा

Transliteration Rāhumudrā

Additional Name *Swarbhanu*

* **Description** *Rahu Mudra* is a joint-hand gesture (*samyukta hasta*) used by performing artists. It is found in the traditional set of the nine planets (*Nava-Graha Hastas*) as described in the *Abhinaya Darpana*. In Hindu mythology, *Rahu* is the severed head of an *asura* (demon) that swallows the sun or moon, thus causing eclipses. He is depicted in Indian art as a serpent with no body, riding a chariot drawn by eight black horses.

* **Technique** Assume *Sarpashirsha Mudra* (p.213) with your left hand and *Suchi Mudra* (p.240) with your right hand. Place your hands in front of your chest. Evoke a cruel gaze.

* **Application** To denote the ascending (north) lunar node, *Rahu*.

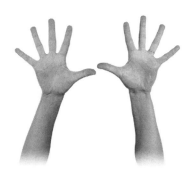

English "demon"

Devanagari रावणमुद्रा

Transliteration Rāvaṇamudrā

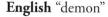 **Description** *Ravana Mudra* is a joint-hand gesture (*samyukta hasta*) common to the dance tradition. In the *Abhinaya Darpana*, it is noted as one of the gestures that indicate "famous emperors and heroes."

Technique Hold the hands with palms facing outward above your shoulders, near your face. Spread your fingers wide and rapidly apply a subtle shake to the hands as you move the hands out to your sides.

Application Used by performing artists to denote the *rakshasa* (demon) *Ravana*, and other wild and ferocious characters.

RECHITA MUDRA
रेचितमुद्रा

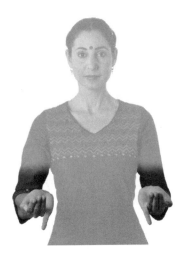

English "emptied"

Devanagari रेचितमुद्रा

Transliteration Recitamudrā

※ **Description** *Rechita Mudra* is a joint-hand dance gesture (*samyukta hasta*) noted in the *Natya Shastra* and *Abhinaya Darpana*. The patron deity associated is *Yaksharaja*.

※ **Technique** Assume *Hamsapaksha Mudra* (p.95) with each hand. Hold the hands waist height, palms facing up, in front of your body.

※ **Application** Used by performing artists to display a painted panel or precious art. Move your hands in an arc-like motion to denote the motion of holding a young child.

रुद्रमुद्रा

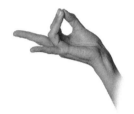

English "roaring," "howling," or "lord of wind and storm"

Devanagari रुद्रमुद्रा

Transliteration Rudramudrā

- **Description** *Rudra Mudra* is a single-hand gesture (*asamyukta hasta*) used in the yogic tradition to open *Manipura Chakra* (the navel center), strengthen digestion, and improve overall vitality.

- **Technique** Join the tips of the index finger, ring finger, and thumb. Extend the middle and little fingers.

- **Application** In a comfortable seated position, form the mudra with each hand. Place the hands on the thighs, palms facing up. Bring your attention to the abdomen, visualizing a golden-red orb of light at your navel growing brighter with each breath. Hold for 5 to 45 minutes. This mudra may also be practiced while walking, standing, or reclining.

- **Benefits** Improves digestion, assimilation, and elimination, regulates body weight, addresses organ prolapses, heals dizziness, sluggishness, and exhaustion.

NOTE *Rudra* is identified as a pre-Vedic deity associated with storms, fire, wildness, ferocity, fertility, cattle, and other domestic animals. Eventually, the name *Rudra* came to represent the fierce aspect of *Shiva*. In post-Vedic times, the names *Rudra* and *Shiva* are often used interchangeably.

RUPA MUDRA

रूपमुद्रा

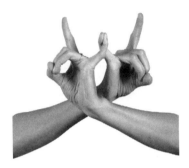

English "form" or "appearance"

Devanagari रूपमुद्रा

Transliteration Rūpamudrā

- **Description** *Rupa Mudra* is a joint-hand gesture (*samyukta hasta*) common to the Buddhist *Vajrayana* tradition. It is usually held by a priest while performing specific rites or rituals, and may often be accompanied by a mantra.

- **Technique** Raise the hand in front of the chest, with the palms facing each other. Cross the wrists, with the left hand in front. Interlock the little fingers. Bend the middle and ring fingers, covering the nails with the pad of the thumb. Extend the index fingers upward.

- **Application** Usually performed to represent or evoke the form of a particular deity or protector.

NOTE Since this mudra is used in the context of ritual, it is not normally associated with particular healing benefits for the individual (although the rituals themselves often have beneficial implications for the community in which they are performed).

सहस्रारमुद्रा

English "thousand-petalled lotus"

Devanagari सहस्रारमुद्रा

Transliteration Sahasrāramudrā

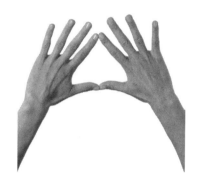

❋ **Description** *Sahasrara Mudra* is a joint-hand gesture (*samyukta hasta*) used in the yogic tradition to access the connection between heaven (sun, moon, stars, and planets) and human beings. This gesture relates to the *Sahasrara Chakra* (crown center) and increases awareness of the spiritual dimension of life and the insight/experience of the interdependent nature of all things.

❋ **Technique** Join the tips of the index fingers and thumbs to form a diamond shape with the hands.

❋ **Application** This mudra may be practiced standing or seated, or in any position, as long as the top of the head is pointing toward the sky. Hold the mudra about 6 inches over your head. Relax the shoulders and breathe naturally. Feel as if you are receiving a shower of light from above. Let this cool light wash through your body from head to toe. Hold for 5 to 20 minutes. Multiple sets per day may be practiced.

❋ **Benefits** Improves brain function, reduces headaches, increases concentration, stimulates the pituitary and pineal glands (benefiting all of the endocrine glands), nourishes the hair, activates the body's self-healing power, calms the spirit, induces the feeling of connection with all life.

NOTE Practicing outdoors under the open sky is a great way to experience this mudra. During daylight hours, when the sun is not too intense, hold the mudra overhead and feel the gentle warmth of the sun illuminate the body from head to toe. Do not practice in direct sunlight between 10 am and 2 pm. At night, you may practice under the light of the moon and stars, feeling the "healing light of heaven" cleanse and heal the body from head to toe.

Samdamsha Mudra

संदंशमुद्रा

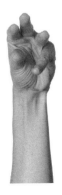

English "biting," "stinging," or "clinging"

Devanagari संदंशमुद्रा

Transliteration Saṁdaṁśamudrā

❋ **Description** *Samdamsha Mudra* is the twenty-fifth hand gesture of the twenty-eight single-hand mudras (*asamyukta hastas*) as described in the *Abhinaya Darpana*. It is also noted in the *Natya Shastra*. According to mythology, this mudra originated from the goddess *Sarasvati* when she held the rosary (*mala*) in her hand. The associated sage is *Visvavasu*, race is *Vidyadhara*, color is white, and patron deity is *Valmiki*.

❋ **Technique** This mudra requires motion. The starting position is identical to *Padmakosha Mudra* (p.180). Maintaining a hollow palm, open and close all five fingers repeatedly.

❋ **Application** Primarily used by performing artists to create context and express emotional states or specific actions. *Viniyoga*: *Udara* ("stomach" or "generosity"); *Balidhana* ("sacrificial offerings"); *Vrana* ("wound"); *Kita* ("insect"); *Maha-bhaya* ("great fear"); *Archana* ("worship"); *Pancha-samkhayam* ("number five"). Additional usages denote: tooth, small bud, singing, *lasya* dance (feminine expression), brief explanation, scales, line, examining, truth, saying "no," saying "a little," moment, listening, poison, slowness, bug, or fly.

NOTE A variation of this mudra is performed with the middle finger extended upward.

Samdamsha Mukula Mudra

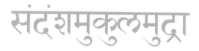
संदंशमुकुलमुद्रा

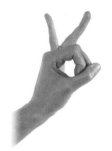

English "grasping bud"

Devanagari संदंशमुकुलमुद्रा

Transliteration Saṃdaṃśamukulamudrā

* **Description** *Samdamsha Mukula Mudra* is a single-hand gesture (*asamyukta hasta*) common to the dance tradition. In the *Abhinaya Darpana*, it is noted as one of the gestures that indicate "flying creatures."

* **Technique** Cover the nails of the index and middle finger with the pad of thumb. Extend the ring and little fingers upward and keep them separated. Flutter your hands to express the movement of a bird.

* **Application** Used in the dance tradition to denote a crow.

SAMPUTA MUDRA I

सम्पुटमुद्रा

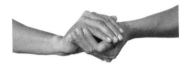

English "bud" or "vessel"

Devanagari सम्पुटमुद्रा

Transliteration Sampuṭamudrā

- **Description** *Samputa Mudra I* is the fourteenth hand gesture of the twenty-four joint-hand mudras (*samyukta hastas*) as described in the *Abhinaya Darpana.*

- **Technique** Cup your hands and join them together palm to palm. Maintain space in the center, as if holding something fragile. Hold the hands about 6 inches in front of your body.

- **Application** Used by performing artists to indicate a casket or a box, as well as to imply the act of concealing things ("*vasthvachada*").

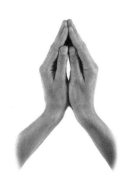

English "bud" or "vessel"

Devanagari सम्पुटमुद्रा

Transliteration Sampuṭamudrā

Additional Name *Kapota*

❋ **Description** *Samputa Mudra II* is a joint-hand gesture (*samyukta hasta*) common to the yoga tradition. It is found in the *Yoga Tattva Mudra Vijnana* form, and is one of the traditional thirty-two *Gayatri Mudras*, specifically the second gesture in the sub-set of twenty-four mudras practiced before meditation or recitation of the *Gayatri Mantra*.

❋ **Technique** Join the tips of all of the fingers. Then, bring the heels of the hands together, so the thumbs rest side by side. Keep the center of the palms hollow, maintaining open space between the hands.

❋ **Application** In a comfortable seated position, hold the mudra in front of the heart center. Relax the shoulders and chest, and breathe naturally. Bring your attention to the space between your hands. Hold this space delicately, as if carrying a baby bird. Hold for 5 to 30 minutes.

❋ **Benefits** Balances all Five Elements, benefits the heart and lungs, reduces mental and emotional suffering, serves as a gateway to directly experiencing exquisite openness, our own Original Nature.

SANKIRNA MUDRA
संकीर्णमुद्रा

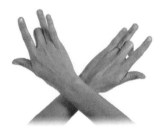

English "cow"

Devanagari संकीर्णमुद्रा

Transliteration Saṁkīrṇamudrā

* **Description** *Sankirna Mudra* is a joint-hand gesture (*samyukta hasta*) common to the dance tradition. It is listed as one of the gestures that indicate "wild animals" in the *Abhinaya Darpana*.

* **Technique** Cross the hands at the wrists, with the palms facing away from you. Bend the middle finger 90 degrees at the second joint, and keep the remaining fingers extended.

* **Application** Used by performing artists to denote a cow.

सपत्निमुद्रा

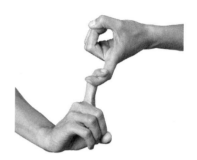

English "co-wife"

Devanagari सपत्निमुद्रा

Transliteration Sapatnimudrā

IMAGE I

✷ **Description** *Sapatni Mudra* is a joint-hand gesture (*samyukta hasta*) used by performing artists. It is found in the traditional set of the eleven relationships (*Bandava Hastas*) as described in the *Abhinaya Darpana*. It indicates co-wife.

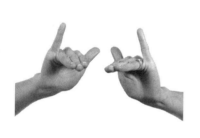

✷ **Technique** This is a progression of two hand gestures performed one after the other. First, assume *Pasha Mudra* (p.185) with both hands (Image I). Then, transition to *Mrigashirsha Mudra* (p.158) with both hands (Image II), and place them on your belly.

✷ **Application** This gesture denotes a co-wife, a wife who has to cope with the relational challenges of sharing a household with other wives.

IMAGE II

SARASVATI MUDRA

सरस्वतीमुद्रा

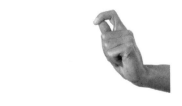

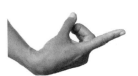

English "goddess of art and knowledge"

Devanagari सरस्वतीमुद्रा

Transliteration Sarasvatīmudrā

Additional names *Bharati, Vagdevi*

   Description *Sarasvati Mudra* is a joint-hand gesture (*samyukta hasta*) used by performing artists. It is found in the traditional set of sixteen *Deva Hastas*, denoting Hindu gods and goddesses as described in the *Abhinaya Darpana*. It indicates the form and character of the Hindu deity *Sarasvati*.[39]

   Technique Assume *Kapittha Mudra* (p.106) with your left hand, and *Suchi Mudra* (p.240) with your right hand. Hold the left hand in front of the left shoulder with the index finger of your right hand pointing toward your left hand.

   Application Used to indicate *Sarasvati*, the Hindu goddess of knowledge, music, art, science, and technology; consort of *Brahma*.

NOTE There are several combinations of mudras used to express the various traits and emblems of *Sarasvati Devi*. The one indicated here appears to be the most common.

SARPASHIRSHA MUDRA

सर्पशीर्षमुद्रा

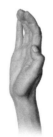

English "serpent head"

Devanagari सर्पशीर्षमुद्रा

Transliteration Sarpaśīrṣamudrā

* **Description** *Sarpashirsha Mudra* is the sixteenth hand gesture of the twenty-eight single-hand mudras (*asamyukta hastas*) as described in the *Abhinaya Darpana*. It is also noted in the *Natya Shastra*. According to mythology, this mudra originated from *Vishnu*, who used it while assuming the form of *Vamana* to protect the *Devas* against *Bali*.[40] The associated sage is *Vasava*, race is *Deva*, color is yellow, and patron deity is *Shiva*.

* **Technique** Raise the hand with the fingers together and palm facing forward. Round the fingers slightly to form the shape of a snake hood.

* **Application** Primarily used by performing artists to create context and express emotional states or specific actions. *Viniyoga*: *Chandana* ("sandal paste"); *Bhujaga* ("snake"); *Mandra* ("low pitch"); *Prokshana* ("sprinkling"); *Poshana* ("nourishing"); *Devasya-udakadhaneshu* ("offering water to god"); *Gaja-kumbhayoh Aspahala* ("flapping of elephant ears"); *Mallanam Bhujasthana* ("wrestler's arms"). Additional usages denote: rouge, mud, doing *pranayama* (breathing practice), washing the face, charity, fondling, milk, saffron flower, bashfulness, concealing a child, image or idol, clinging, saying "very true," and holding a woman's breast.

SHAKATA MUDRA I

शकटमुद्रा

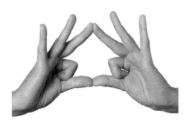

English "cart" or "carriage"

Devanagari शकटमुद्रा

Transliteration Śakaṭamudrā

⁕ **Description** *Shakata Mudra I* is the eleventh hand gesture of the twenty-four joint-hand mudras (*samyukta hastas*) as described in the *Abhinaya Darpana*.

⁕ **Technique** Roll the index finger into the base of the thumb on each hand. Extend the remaining fingers, connecting the tips of the thumbs and middle fingers.

⁕ **Application** Used by performing artists to denote *rakshasas* ("demons"). In the dynamic version, the two hands are separated and moved toward the sides of the head.

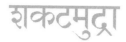

English "cart" or "carriage"

Devanagari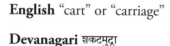

Transliteration Śakaṭamudrā

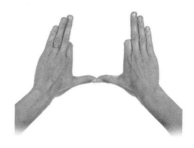

IMAGE I

✸ **Description** *Shakata Mudra II* is a joint-hand gesture (*samyukta hasta*) common to the yoga tradition. It is found in the *Yoga Tattva Mudra Vijnana* form, and is one of the traditional thirty-two *Gayatri Mudras*, specifically the twelfth gesture in the sub-set of twenty-four mudras practiced before meditation or recitation of the *Gayatri Mantra*.

✸ **Technique** With the palms facing down, lightly join the tips of the thumbs. Variation 1: Extend the index finger forward and curl the other fingers in toward the palms (Image I). Variation 2: Bend the index finger 90 degrees at the middle joint, and extend the remaining fingers (Image II).

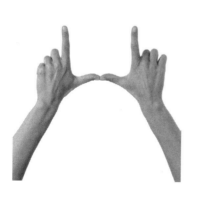

✸ **Application** In a comfortable seated position, hold the mudra in front of the solar plexus. Relax the chest, shoulders, and belly. Breathe naturally and hold for 5 to 30 minutes.

✸ **Benefits** Strengthens the immune system, facilitates breathing in the lower lobes of the lungs, improves concentration, benefits the large intestine.

IMAGE II

SHAKTI MUDRA
शक्तिमुद्रा

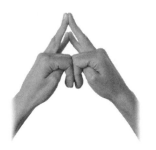

English "creative force" or "goddess of vital energy"

Devanagari शक्तिमुद्रा

Transliteration Śaktimudrā

* **Description** *Shakti Mudra* is a joint-hand gesture (*samyukta hasta*) used in the yoga tradition to induce sleep and relax the organs and musculature of the pelvis.

* **Technique** With the palms facing each other, join the tips of the ring and little fingers. Fold the thumbs into the palms and cover them with the index and middle fingers.

* **Application** In a comfortable seated position, hold the mudra in front of the heart center. Soften the belly and breathe naturally. Bring attention to your pelvis, noticing the sensations and emotion that arise. Without judgment or criticism, let your experience unfold spontaneously. Whatever arises during this practice, treat it with great care and tenderness. Hold for 5 to 45 minutes.

* **Benefits** Calms the mind, relaxes the body, induces sound sleep, reduces cramping of lower abdominal organs (especially useful for relieving menstrual cramps), releases pelvic tension, heals physical and emotional trauma associated with unconscious sex and/or sexual abuse, opens the doorway to receptivity and intimacy, serves as a powerful connection to the divine feminine, the lunar rhythm, tides, and the myriad other cycles of nature.

SHANI MUDRA

शनिमुद्रा

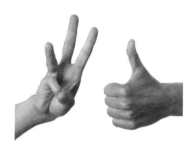

English "planet Saturn"

Devanagari शनिमुद्रा

Transliteration Śanimudrā

Additional names *Sanaischara, Manda, Sthitra, Souri*

* **Description** *Shani Mudra* is a joint-hand gesture (*samyukta hasta*) used by performing artists. It is found in the traditional set of the nine planets (*Nava-Graha Hastas*) as described in the *Abhinaya Darpana*. It indicates the character of the planet Saturn.

* **Technique** Assume *Shikhara Mudra* (p.225) with your left hand and *Trishula Mudra* (p.254) with your right hand. Place the hands in front of your chest and stand in *sama* position (straight and elongated posture). Assume a menacing gaze.

* **Application** To denote the planet Saturn. This mudra, in its dynamic form, requires movement of the hands in a winding manner in front of the face.

SHANKHA MUDRA I

शङ्खमुद्रा

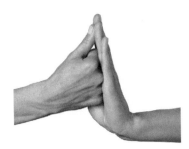

English "conch shell"

Devanagari शङ्खमुद्रा

Transliteration Śaṅkhamudrā

﹡ **Description** *Shankha Mudra I* is the twelfth hand gesture of the twenty-four joint-hand mudras (*samyukta hastas*) as described in the *Abhinaya Darpana*.

﹡ **Technique** Grasp the left thumb with the right hand. Bring the hands together, with the tip of the right thumb touching the tips of the left index, middle, and ring fingers.

﹡ **Application** Used by performing artists to signify the *Shankha* ("conch shell"), which often denotes *Vishnu*. It is one of the sacred emblems of the Hindu god of preservation (*Vishnu*). *Vishnu* holds the *Shankha* in his upper left hand, which represents his power to create and maintain the universe.

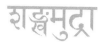

English "conch shell"

Devanagari शङ्खमुद्रा

Transliteration Śaṅkhamudrā

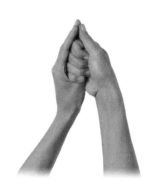

❁ **Description** *Shankha Mudra II* is a joint-hand gesture (*samyukta hasta*) common to the yoga tradition. It is found in the *Yoga Tattva Mudra Vijnana* form, and is one of the traditional thirty-two *Gayatri Mudras*, specifically the fifth gesture in the sub-set of eight mudras practiced after meditation or recitation of the *Gayatri Mantra*.

❁ **Technique** Grasp the left thumb with the right hand. Bring the hands together, with the tip of the right thumb touching the tips of the left index, middle, and ring fingers.

❁ **Application** In a comfortable seated position, raise the mudra in front of the heart. Relax the shoulders and belly, and breathe naturally. Lengthen the spine, and become very still and quiet. Listen intently to the silence. Hold for 5 to 45 minutes.

❁ **Benefits** Improves the voice, helps reduce speech defects such as stuttering, calms the mind, improves concentration, nourishes the kidneys and sexual glands (testes and ovaries), benefits the hair and bones, has a special connection with the navel center, thereby improving digestion and increasing appetite.

Shankhasura Mudra

शङ्खसुरमुद्रा

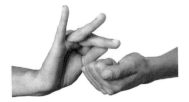

English "name of a demon"

Devanagari शङ्खसुरमुद्रा

Transliteration Śaṅkhasuramudrā

- **Description** *Shankhasura Mudra* is a joint-hand gesture (*samyukta hasta*) common to the dance tradition.

- **Technique** Form a fist with the left hand (with the thumb resting against the outside of the index finger), and turn the hand palm facing up. With the right hand, form *Bhramara Mudra* (p.64). Place your right thumb on top of the left little finger.

- **Application** Used by performing artists to denote a demon.

शङ्खवर्तमुद्रा

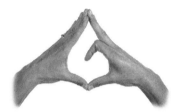

English "conch livelihood"

Devanagari शङ्खवर्तमुद्रा

Transliteration Śaṅkhavartamudrā

❋ **Description** *Shankhavarta Mudra* is a joint-hand gesture (*samyukta hasta*) common to the Buddhist *Vajrayana* tradition. It is a Tantric mudra representing the conch shell, one of the *Ashtamangala*, "eight auspicious symbols," the others being: a parasol, victory banner, golden fish, *dharma* (wheel), knot of wisdom, lotus flower, and treasure vase. These eight symbols represent the eight offerings made by the gods to *Shakyamuni Buddha* after he attained enlightenment.

❋ **Technique** Raise the hands in front of the heart, palms facing each other. Join the tips of all the fingers. Bend the right index finger about 90 degrees at the middle joint.

❋ **Application** In a comfortable seated position, hold the mudra in front of the heart. Relax the chest and shoulders, and breathe naturally. Become very still and quiet, listening to the silence. Hold for 5 to 45 minutes.

❋ **Benefits** Quiets the mind, turns the attention inward, strengthens intuition, serves as a gateway to "hear" the wordless teachings of your own Original Nature.

SHANMUKHA MUDRA I

षण्मुखमुद्रा

 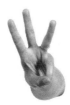

English "deity of war" or "six faces"

Devanagari षण्मुखमुद्रा

Transliteration Śaṇmukhamudrā

Additional names *Kartikeya, Muruga, Kumaraswamy, Subrahmanya, Skanda*

❋ **Description** *Shanmukha Mudra I* is a joint-hand gesture (*samyukta hasta*) used by performing artists. It is found in the traditional set of sixteen *Deva Hastas*, denoting Hindu gods and goddesses as described in the *Abhinaya Darpana*. It indicates the form and character of the Hindu deity *Shanmukha*.[41]

❋ **Technique** Assume *Trishula Mudra* (p.254) with your left hand and *Shikhara Mudra* (p.225) with your right hand. Hold the gestures at shoulder height, pointing upward.

❋ **Application** Used to indicate *Shanmukha*, the Hindu god of war.

NOTE There are several combinations of mudras used to express the various traits and emblems of *Shanmukha Deva*. The one indicated here appears to be the most common.

षण्मुखमुद्रा

English "six faces"

Devanagari षण्मुखमुद्रा

Transliteration Śaṇmukhamudrā

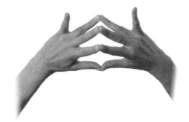

※ **Description** *Shanmukha Mudra II* is a joint-hand gesture (*samyukta hasta*) common to the yoga tradition. It is found in the *Yoga Tattva Mudra Vijnana* form, and is one of the traditional thirty-two *Gayatri Mudras*, specifically the ninth gesture in the sub-set of twenty-four mudras practiced before meditation or recitation of the *Gayatri Mantra*.

※ **Technique** Join the tips of the thumbs, index, middle, and ring fingers. Extend the little fingers forward.

※ **Application** In a comfortable seated position, hold the mudra in front of the solar plexus. Relax the chest, shoulder, and abdomen. Breathe naturally. Hold for 5 to 45 minutes.

※ **Benefits** Activates the body's self-healing power, strengthens the immune system, improves memory, benefits the hair and bones, increases spiritual devotion.

SHANMUKHI MUDRA

षण्मुखीमुद्रा

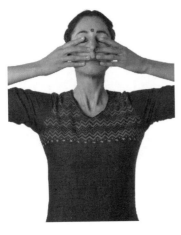

English "six faces" or "six openings"

Devanagari षण्मुखीमुद्रा

Transliteration Ṣaṇmukhīmudrā

✵ **Description** *Shanmukhi Mudra* is a joint-hand gesture (*samyukta hasta*) common to the yoga tradition. It is used as a tool to assist the practice of *pratyahara* (interiorization of the senses).

✵ **Technique/Application** Sit in a comfortable position and raise the hands to the level of the head, palms facing your face. Take a deep breath and hold the air in. Close the ears with the thumbs, the eyes with the index fingers, the nostrils with the middle fingers, and the upper and lower lips with the ring and little fingers respectively. Closing the out-flowing of all the senses, look within. Hold the breath as long as you comfortably can without feeling strain or anxiety. Exhale silently and release the mudra. You can repeat up to 36 times. Beyond this, the guidance of a qualified teacher is recommended.

✵ **Benefits** Helps develop concentration, trains the mind to turn inward for meditation and other contemplative practices.

CAUTION Press very gently on the eyelids. Breath retention is contraindicated during pregnancy, recent abdominal surgery, hernia, history of stroke, heart disease, and high blood pressure.

शीखरमुद्रा

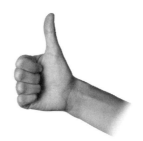

English "spire" or "peak of the mountain"

Devanagari शीखरमुद्रा

Transliteration Śīkharamudrā

Additional Name *Aratrika*

   ❁   **Description** *Shikhara Mudra* is the tenth hand gesture of the twenty-eight single-hand mudras (*asamyukta hastas*) as described in the *Abhinaya Darpana*. It is also noted in the *Natya Shastra,* and in the *Abhinaya Chandrika* as *Aratika*. According to mythology, this mudra originated from *Chandrasekhara* (*Shiva*), when he held Mount Meru with this gesture as his bow. The associated sage is *Jihna*, race is *Gandharva*, color is dusky, and patron deity is the god of love (known by many names such as *Smara, Manmatha, Kama, Madana*).

   ❁   **Technique** From a fist with the thumb extended upward.

   ❁   **Application** Used by performing artists to create context and express emotional states or specific actions. *Viniyoga*: *Madhana* ("god of love"); *Kamuka* ("bow"); *Sthamba* ("pillar"); *Nishchaya* ("resolve"); *Pithrukarmani* ("offerings to ancestors"); *Oshtra* ("lips"); *Pravishtarupa* ("pouring liquid" or "entering"); *Radana* ("teeth"); *Prashna-bhavana* ("questioning"); *Linga* ("masculine principle" or "phallus"); *Nasti-iti-vachana* ("saying no"); *Samarana* ("recollection"); *Abhinaya-anthikam* ("intimate suggestion"); *Kati-bandha-akarshana* ("tightening the waist band"); *Parirambha-vidikrama* ("embracing"); *Dhave* ("husband"); *Gantaninadha* ("sounding a bell"); *Peshane* ("pounding"). Additional usages denote: establishing a family, hero, hill top, friend, cleaning the teeth, fanning one's face, difference, saying "what," drinking water, the number four, enjoying consequences, demure of an amorous girl, bashfulness, bow, heroism, galloping, applying *tilaka*,[42] tying the hair in a top-knot.

SHIVA MUDRA

शिवमुद्रा

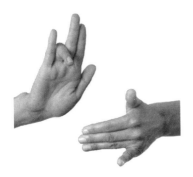

English "god of transformation"

Devanagari शिवमुद्रा

Transliteration Śivamudrā

Additional names *Shambu, Sadashiva, Ishwara, Chandrakeshara, Ardhanarishwara*

※ **Description** *Shiva Mudra* is a joint-hand gesture (*samyukta hasta*) used by performing artists. It is found in the traditional set of sixteen *Deva Hastas*, denoting Hindu gods and goddesses as described in the *Abhinaya Darpana*. It indicates the form and character of the Hindu deity *Shiva*.

※ **Technique** Assume *Mrigashirsha Mudra* (p.158) with your left hand and *Tripataka Mudra* (p.253) with your right hand. The left hand is turned palm facing you, held near the waistline; the right hand is held in front of the right shoulder.

※ **Application** Used to indicate *Shiva*, the Hindu god of transformation. Stand with your feet apart and hold the gestures about 6 inches away from your body.

NOTE There are several combinations of mudras used to express the various traits and emblems of *Shiva*. The one indicated here appears to be the most common.

शिवलिङ्गमुद्रा

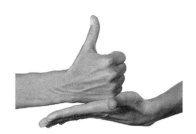

English "masculine creative energy"

Devanagari शिवलिङ्गमुद्रा

Transliteration Śivaliṅgamudrā

* **Description** *Shivalinga Mudra* is the eighth hand gesture of the twenty-four joint-hand mudras (*samyukta hastas*) as described in the *Abhinaya Darpana*.

* **Technique** Assume *Shikhara Mudra* (p.225) with your right hand and *Ardhachandra Mudra* (p.48) with your left hand. Place your right fist on top of your left palm, holding the gesture about 6 inches in front of your body.

* **Application** Primarily used by performing artists to signify *Shiva Lingam*, representing the deity *Shiva*. The *Lingam* is a symbol of male creative energy or the phallus. The *Lingam* also represents the beginning-less and endless *stambha* pillar,[43] symbolizing the infinite nature of *Shiva*.

Shukachanchu Mudra

शुकचञ्चुमुद्रा

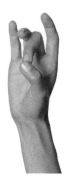

English "parrot's beak"

Devanagari शुकचञ्चुमुद्रा

Transliteration Śukacañcumudrā

Additional Name *Ankusha*

❁ **Description** *Shukachanchu Mudra* is a single-hand mudra (*asamyukta hasta*) common to the dance tradition. It is noted in the *Abhinaya Chandrika*. According to mythology, it originated from the supreme goddess of love and beauty, *Lalita Mahatripurasundari*, depicted as holding her traditional implements: flower arrows, noose, goad, and sugarcane bow.

❁ **Technique** Touch the tip of your middle finger to the tip of the thumb. All other fingers are slightly curled in a graceful and natural manner.

❁ **Application** Used by performing artists to denote the goddess, or a beautiful and graceful woman. Typically applied with the tip of the index finger touching the side of the chin.

शुक्तुण्डमुद्रा

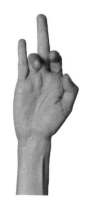

English "parrot's beak"

Devanagari शुक्तुण्डमुद्रा

Transliteration Śukatuṇḍamudrā

* **Description** *Shukatunda Mudra* is the eighth hand gesture of the twenty-eight single-hand mudras (*asamyukta hastas*) as described in the *Abhinaya Darpana*. It is also noted in the *Natya Shastra*. According to mythology, it originated from *Parvati* who used it in a lovers' quarrel with *Sadashiva*. The associated sage is *Dhruvasa*, race is *Bramhana*, color is red, and patron deity is *Marici* (or *Sadashiva*).

* **Technique** With the hand facing away from you, bend the index and ring finger 90 degrees at the second joint. The thumb, middle, and little finger point upward.

* **Application** Primarily used by performing artists to create context and express emotional states or specific actions. *Viniyoga*: *Bana-prayuga* ("shooting an arrow"); *Kuntartha* ("spear"); *Alayasya-smritikarma* ("remembering the past"); *Marmukthyam* ("mystic mood"); *Ugrabhava* ("ferocity"). Additional usages denote: *Brahma*'s weapon, nose, crookedness, change, turning around, proceeding, fighting, crossing, disrespect, lovers' quarrel, opinion, abandonment, gambling dice, throwing a spear, ferocity, and secrecy.

NOTE In the *Hasta Lakshana Deepika*, *Shukatunda Mudra* is noted as a different hand formation, identical to *Tamrachudha Mudra* of the *Abhinaya Darpana*.

SHUKRA MUDRA

शुक्रमुद्रा

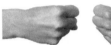

English "planet Venus" or "pure"

Devanagari शुक्रमुद्रा

Transliteration Śukramudrā

Additional Name *Bhargava*

⊛ **Description** *Shukra Mudra* is a joint-hand gesture (*samyukta hasta*) used by performing artists. It is found in the traditional set of the nine planets (*Nava-Graha Hastas*) as described in the *Abhinaya Darpana*. It indicates the character of the planet Venus.

⊛ **Technique** Form *Mushti Mudra* (p.163) with each hand.

⊛ **Application** Denotes the planet Venus. Traditionally, the left hand is raised and the right is lowered. The head moves up and down quickly and the eyes are half-closed.

शुक्रिमुद्रा

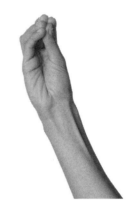

English "virtuous action" or "having purity"

Devanagari शुक्रिमुद्रा

Transliteration Śukrimudrā

❋ **Description** *Shukri Mudra* is a single-hand gesture (*asamyukta hasta*) common to the yoga tradition. It is found in the *Yoga Tattva Mudra Vijnana* form, where it is used to calm the mind and restore vigor.

❋ **Technique** Join the tips of all of the fingers.

❋ **Application** This mudra may be practiced in any position: walking, standing, seated, or lying down. It may be held with one hand, or both hands. For the purposes of deeper restoration and rejuvenation, it is best to practice lying down in *shavasana* (corpse pose). Hold for 5 to 30 minutes.

❋ **Benefits** Balances the Five Elements, bolsters immunity, rejuvenates the organs and blood, soothes the nerves, evokes a peaceful state of mind.

Shunya Mudra

शून्यमुद्रा

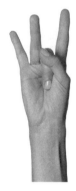

English "emptiness," "zero," "sky," or "hollow reed"

Devanagari शून्यमुद्रा

Transliteration Śūnyamudrā

❁ **Description** *Shunya Mudra* is a single-hand gesture (*asamyukta hasta*) common to the yoga tradition. It is part of the *Yoga Tattva Mudra Vijnana* form, where it is used to improve hearing and benefit the ears.

❁ **Technique** Fold the middle finger into the palm with the tip resting at the base of the thumb. Cover the middle finger with the thumb, and extend the remaining fingers.

❁ **Application** This mudra may be practiced in any position, while walking, standing, seated, or lying down. For a more in-depth experience, sit in a comfortable seated position with the spine erect. Relax the chest and belly, and breathe naturally. Form the mudra with each hand and rest the hands in the lap, palms facing up. Hold for 5 to 30 minutes. For best results in improving hearing, practice 2 to 3 sessions per day.

❁ **Benefits** Improves hearing, reduces ringing in the ears (tinnitus) and earache, decreases vertigo, improves balance.

NOTE *Shunya Mudra* is especially useful during travel. With air travel, it helps the ears adjust to the changing pressure during take-off and landing. During water and land travel, it helps prevent motion sickness.

CAUTION Short-term use of this mudra for acute situations such as travel is perfectly safe. However, regular long-term practice of this mudra is not recommended. Once hearing has improved, or desired effects have been realized, it is best to discontinue regular practice of *Shunya Mudra*.

SHVASHRU MUDRA

श्वश्रूमुद्रा

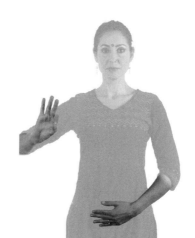

English "mother-in-law"

Devanagari श्वश्रूमुद्रा

Transliteration Śvaśrūmudrā

* **Description** *Shvashru Mudra* is a joint-hand gesture (*samyukta hasta*) used by performing artists. It is found in the traditional set of the eleven relationships (*Bandava Hastas*) as described in the *Abhinaya Darpana.* It indicates mother-in-law.

* **Technique** Assume *Ardhachandra Mudra* (p.48) with your left hand and place it on your stomach (this is the *stri* "feminine" hand). Form *Hamsasya Mudra* (p.96) with your right hand and hold it in front of your chest or throat.

* **Application** Used by performing artists to denote mother-in-law.

SHVASHURA MUDRA

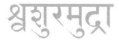

English "father-in-law"

Devanagari श्वशुरमुद्रा

Transliteration Śvaśuramudrā

- **Description** *Shvashura Mudra* is a joint-hand gesture (*samyukta hasta*) used by performing artists. It is found in the traditional set of the eleven relationships (*Bandava Hastas*) as described in the *Abhinaya Darpana*. It indicates father-in-law.

- **Technique** Assume *Hamsasya Mudra* (p.96) with your left hand and *Shikhara Mudra* (p.225) with your right hand. Hold both hands in front of your body.

- **Application** Used by performing artists to denote father-in-law.

Simha Mudra

सिंहमुद्रा

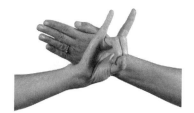

English "lion"

Devanagari सिंहमुद्रा

Transliteration Simhamudrā

- ❋ **Description** *Simha Mudra* is a joint-hand gesture (*samyukta hasta*) common to the dance tradition. In the *Abhinaya Darpana*, it is noted as one of the gestures that indicate "wild animals."

- ❋ **Technique** With the right hand facing away from you, cover the nails of the middle and ring fingers with the pad of the thumb. Hold the left hand with the fingers collected, palm facing you. Touch the backs of the two hands together.

- ❋ **Application** Used in the dance tradition to denote a lion.

SIMHAKRANTA MUDRA

सिंहक्रान्तमुद्रा

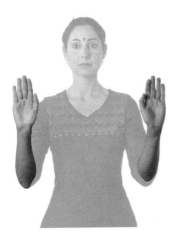

English "lion nature"

Devanagari सिंहक्रान्तमुद्रा

Transliteration Siṁhakrāntamudrā

Additional Name *Singhakranta*

❋ **Description** *Simhakranta Mudra* is a joint-hand gesture (*samyukta hasta*) common to the yoga tradition. It is found in the *Yoga Tattva Mudra Vijnana* form, and is one of the traditional thirty-two *Gayatri Mudras*, specifically the twenty-first gesture in the sub-set of twenty-four mudras practiced before meditation or recitation of the *Gayatri Mantra*. The lion represents one of the various forms *Vishnu* took to benefit Earth. It denotes courage, majesty, and virtue.

❋ **Technique** Raise the hands in front of the shoulders with the palms facing forward, and fingers extending up.

❋ **Application** In a comfortable seated position, lengthen the spine, relax the shoulders, and breathe naturally. Hold the mudra with the elbows pointing downward and the hands relaxed. Hold for 5 to 30 minutes.

❋ **Benefits** Activates the body's self-healing power, balances the immune system, increases courage (especially in the practice of self-honesty), increases devotion and loyalty.

सिंहमुखमुद्रा

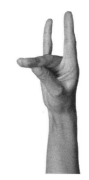

English "lion face"

Devanagari सिंहमुखमुद्रा

Transliteration Siṁhamukhamudrā

Additional Names *Singhamukha, Mragi*

◉ **Description** *Simhamukha Mudra* is the eighteenth hand gesture of the twenty-eight single-hand mudras (*asamyukta hastas*) as described in the *Abhinaya Darpana.*

✳ **Technique** Touch the pad of the thumb to the top joint creases of the middle and ring fingers. Extend the index and little fingers upward.

✳ **Application** Primarily used by performing artists to create context and express emotional states or specific actions. *Viniyoga: Vidruma* ("coral"); *Mauktika* ("pearl"); *Sugandha* ("fragrance"); *Alaka-sampsarsa* ("stroking hair"); *Akarnane* ("hearing"); *Prushati* ("water drop"); *Hridi-samsthitah moksha-artha* ("salvation"); *Homa* ("fire ritual"); *Shasha* ("rabbit"); *Gaja* ("elephant"); *Dharba-chalana* ("waving kusha grass"); *Padma-damani* (" lotus garland"); *Simha-anana* ("lion's face"); *Vaidy-paka-sodhana* ("testing medicine preparation").

NOTE *Simhamukha Mudra* is also known as *Mragi Mudra* in the yoga tradition and is found in the *Yoga Tattva Mudra Vijnana* form.

SINDHUVARA MUDRA
सिन्धुवरमुद्रा

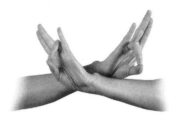

English "type of tree"

Devanagari सिन्धुवरमुद्रा

Transliteration Sindhuvaramudrā

* **Description** *Sindhuvara Mudra* is a joint-hand gesture (*samyukta hasta*) common to the dance tradition. It is listed as one of the mudras indicating "trees" in the *Abhinaya Darpana*.

* **Technique** With the palms facing away from you, form *Mayura Mudra* (p.154) with each hand and cross the wrists.

* **Application** Used in the dance tradition to denote the *sindhuvara* tree.

स्नुषामुद्रा

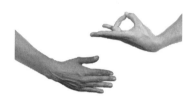

English "daughter-in-law"

Devanagari स्नुषामुद्रा

Transliteration Snuṣāmudrā

※ **Description** *Snusha Mudra* is a joint-hand gesture (*samyukta hasta*) used by performing artists. It is found in the traditional set of the eleven relationships (*Bandava Hastas*) as described in the *Abhinaya Darpana*. It indicates daughter-in-law.

※ **Technique** Form *Mayura Mudra* (p.154) with your left hand, palm facing upward, and *Mrigashirsha Mudra* (p.158) with your right hand, and place it on the stomach (this is the *stri* "feminine" hand).

※ **Application** This gesture denotes daughter-in-law.

SUCHI MUDRA
सुचिमुद्रा

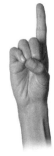

English "needle"

Devanagari सुचिमुद्रा

Transliteration Sucimudrā

Additional Name *Nirdeshika*

❈ **Description** *Suchi Mudra* is the thirteenth hand gesture of the twenty-eight single-hand mudras (*asamyukta hastas*) as described in the *Abhinaya Darpana*. It is also noted in the *Natya Shastra* and in the *Abhinaya Chandrika* as *Nirdeshika*. According to mythology, the mudra originated from *Brahma*, when he declared, "I'm matchless." The associated sage is *Surya*, the sun, race is *Deva*, color is white, and patron deity is *Vishvakarma*.[44]

❈ **Technique** Extend the index finger while keeping the remaining fingers collected under the tip of the thumb.

❈ **Application** Primarily used by performing artists to create context and express emotional states or specific actions. *Viniyoga: Eka-artha* ("denoting number one"); *Parabrahma-bhavana* ("supreme being"); *Shata* ("denoting hundred"); *Ravi* ("sun"); *Nagaryam* ("city"); *Lokartham* ("world"); *Tatha-iti-vachanam* ("to say 'like that'"); *Yat-shabde tat-sabde* ("asking this or that?"); *Vyajana-artha* ("solitude"); *Tharjana* ("threatening"); *Karshya* ("growing thin"); *Shalaka* ("rod"); *Vapushi* ("body"); *Ascharya* ("astonishment"); *Venibhavana* ("braid of hair"); *Chatra* ("umbrella"); *Samartha* ("capability"); *Panau* ("hand"); *Romalayam* ("line of hair," such as eyebrow or on the abdomen); *Bherivadana* ("beating a drum"); *Kulala-chakra-bramana* ("potter's wheel"); *Rathanga-mandala* ("chariot wheel"); *Vivechana* ("pros and cons"); *Dina-anta* ("end of the day"). Also used to denote: praising, telling truth, pointing to distant place, life, walking in front, lotus stalk, sunrise and sunset, arrow, handle, listening, yearning for the beloved, recollection, nose, beak, and vision.

सुचिधरमुद्रा

English "edge of the needle" or "holding a needle"

Devanagari सुचिधरमुद्रा

Transliteration Sucidharamudrā

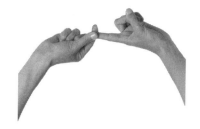

❋ **Description** *Suchidhara Mudra* is a joint-hand gesture (*samyukta hasta*) mentioned in the *Odissi Dance Pathfinder Vol. II.*

❋ **Technique** Form *Suchi Mudra* (p.240) with the left hand. With the thumb and index finger of the right hand, firmly hold the left index finger while keeping the other fingers tucked into the palm. Hold the gesture above the head, framing your face.

❋ **Application** *Suchidhara Mudra* is utilized to highlight the *lasya* (feminine grace) of the dancer, and is frequently used by dancers in *Pallavis* ("pure dance" forms). It is the hand gesture of the *chari* (transitional phrase) titled *Bishama Sanchara.*

SUMUKHA MUDRA

सुमुखमुद्रा

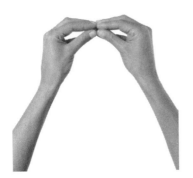

English "good/pleasant face"

Devanagari सुमुखमुद्रा

Transliteration Sumukhamudrā

❁ **Description** *Sumukha Mudra* is a joint-hand gesture (*samyukta hasta*) common to the yoga tradition. It is found in the *Yoga Tattva Mudra Vijnana* form, and is one of the traditional thirty-two *Gayatri Mudras*, specifically the first gesture in the sub-set of twenty-four mudras practiced before meditation or recitation of the *Gayatri Mantra*.

❁ **Technique** Join the tips of all of the fingers of each hand. Touch the two hands together at the fingertips.

❁ **Application** In a comfortable seated position, lengthen the spine, and relax the shoulders, chest, and belly. Hold the mudra in front of the solar plexus (below the sternum). Breathe naturally and hold for 5 to 30 minutes.

❁ **Benefits** Balances left and right sides of the body, harmonizes all Five Elements, activates the body's self-healing power, benefits the tendons and bones, increases concentration power, builds devotion and spiritual resolve.

SURABHI MUDRA

सुरभिमुद्रा

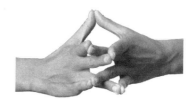

English "cow"

Devanagari सुरभिमुद्रा

Transliteration Surabhimudrā

Additional Name *Dhenu*

※ **Description** *Surabhi Mudra* is an intricate joint-hand gesture (*samyukta hasta*) common to the yoga tradition. It is found in the *Yoga Tattva Mudra Vijnana* form, and is one of the traditional thirty-two *Gayatri Mudras*, specifically the first gesture in the sub-set of eight mudras practiced after meditation or recitation of the *Gayatri Mantra*.

※ **Technique** Join the palms together in front of the chest. Cross the left middle finger behind the right. Join the tip of the left middle finger with the tip of the right index, and the tip of the right middle finger with the tip of the left index. Cross the left ring finger behind the right. Touch the tip of the left ring finger to the right little finger, and the tip of the right ring finger to the tip of the left little finger. Join the tips of the thumbs.

※ **Application** In a comfortable seated position, lengthen the spine, and relax the shoulders, chest, and belly. Raise the mudra to the level of the heart. Breathe naturally and hold for 5 to 30 minutes.

※ **Benefits** Balances *Vata Dosha* (see Appendix A), treats cough and bile disorders, improves memory, reduces inflammation (especially related to rheumatism), awakens empathy, reduces ego grasping, gives insight into one's hidden gifts and talents (and how these can be used to benefit all beings), increases devotion and spiritual radiance.

Surya Mudra I
सूर्यमुद्रा

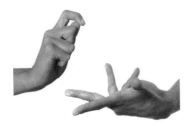

English "sun god"

Devanagari सूर्यमुद्रा

Transliteration Sūryamudrā

Additional names *Divakara, Arka, Bhanu, Aditya, Bhaskara*

※ **Description** *Surya Mudra I* is a joint-hand gesture (*samyukta hasta*) used by performing artists. It is found in the traditional set of sixteen *Deva Hastas*, denoting Hindu gods and goddesses as described in the *Abhinaya Darpana*. It indicates the form and character of the Hindu deity *Surya*.

※ **Technique** Form *Kapittha Mudra* (p.106) with your right hand and *Alapadma Mudra* (p.41) with your left hand. Place both hands around chest level and stand in *sama* position (straight and elongated posture). Assume a pleasant gaze.

※ **Application** To denote the sun.

NOTE In addition to this general mudra to indicate the sun, there are other hand formations mentioned in the *Abhinaya Darpana* that denote the rising sun, midday sun, and setting sun.[45]

सूर्यमुद्रा

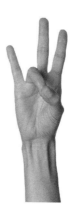

English "sun"

Devanagari सूर्यमुद्रा

Transliteration Sūryamudrā

❋ **Description** *Surya Mudra II* is a single-hand gesture (*asamyukta hasta*) common to the yoga tradition. It is found in the *Yoga Tattva Mudra Vijnana* form, where it is used for weight loss, depression, and to improve digestion.

❋ **Technique** Cover the nail of the ring finger with the pad of the thumb and extend the remaining fingers, keeping them relaxed.

❋ **Application** This mudra may be practiced in any position: while walking, sitting, standing, or lying down. For increased benefit, practice first thing in the morning on an empty stomach. Sit in a comfortable seated position with the spine erect. Form the mudra with each hand and place the hands on the thighs, palms up. Relax the chest, shoulders, and belly, and breathe naturally. Relax in stillness. Hold for 5 to 45 minutes.

❋ **Benefits** Burns excess fat, improves digestion, reduces cholesterol, detoxifies the body, increases body temperature, reduces sluggishness, mental fogginess, and depression.

NOTE *Surya Mudra II* will have increased benefits for improving digestive function if practiced while sitting in *Vajrasana* (thunderbolt pose). Kneel on the floor with the inner thighs together. Rest the buttocks on the heels and settle the weight down. Then, follow the directions above.

Svadhisthana Chakra Mudra
स्वाधिष्ठानचक्रमुद्रा

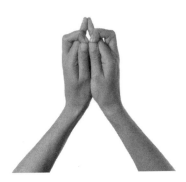

English "self abode"

Devanagari स्वाधिष्ठानचक्रमुद्रा

Transliteration Svādhiṣṭhānacakramudrā

❋ **Description** *Svadhishthana Chakra Mudra* is an intricate joint-hand gesture (*samyukta hasta*) used in Tantric Yoga and Japanese martial arts to open the *Svadhishthana Chakra* (the pelvic center) and increase the ability to adapt to changing circumstances.

❋ **Technique** Cross the middle fingers over the index fingers on each hand. Interlace the ring and little fingers, folding them into the palm. Touch the tips of the index fingers together and bring the thumbs up to the tips of the middle fingers. Press the heels of the hands together, with the sides of the thumbs touching.

❋ **Application** In a comfortable seated position, lengthen the spine and relax the shoulders, chest, and belly. Place the tip of the tongue against the upper palate, and soften the inside of the mouth. Rest the mudra against your pubic bone, and breathe naturally. Hold for 5 to 45 minutes.

❋ **Benefits** Increases ability to adapt to change, opens creativity and the ability to spontaneously respond to any situation, increases capacity for intimacy with self, others, and the environment, benefits the reproductive system, improves sexual health and fertility, tonifies the blood.

Note This mudra requires considerable flexibility in the fingers. Go easy at first, practicing for shorter durations (a minute or two is plenty), until the fingers become accustomed to the position. Once your hands feel comfortable holding the mudra, you may practice for longer periods to experience the deeper dimensions of this powerful mudra.

Caution Contraindicated during pregnancy, unless practiced under the guidance of an expert instructor.

Svastika Mudra
स्वस्तिकमुद्रा

English "crossed"

Devanagari स्वस्तिकमुद्रा

Transliteration Svastikamudrā

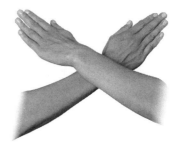

❉ **Description** *Svastika Mudra* is the fourth hand gesture of the twenty-four joint-hand mudras (*samyukta hastas*) as described in the *Abhinaya Darpana*. It is also noted in the *Natya Shastra*. The patron deity associated with it is *Bharati*.

❉ **Technique** Cross the wrists with the palms resting on the upper chest. Keep the fingers extended and collected, palms flat (as in *Pataka Mudra*).

❉ **Application** Primarily used by performing artists to create context and express emotional states or specific actions. *Viniyoga*: *Makara-artha* ("crocodile"); *Bhaya-vada* ("timid speech"); *Vivada* ("dispute"); Kirtana ("praise"); *Svastikaiya* ("crossing"). The dynamic move of separating the hands apart represents movement of clouds, jungles, oceans, the earth, and vastness in general.

NOTE In the *Natya Shastra*, a different version of this mudra is noted, where *Arala* is used in place of *Pataka*.

Svastikamukha Mudra

स्वस्तिकमुखमुद्रा

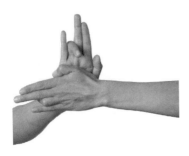

English "cross face"

Devanagari स्वस्तिकमुखमुद्रा

Transliteration Svastikamukhamudrā

❀ **Description** *Svastikamukha Mudra* is a joint-hand gesture (*samyukta hasta*) noted in the *Natya Shastra* and *Abhinaya Darpana*. The patron deity associated with it is *Guha*.[46]

❀ **Technique** Form *Tripataka Mudra* (p.253) with each hand. The right hand is held to the outside of the right shoulder, palm facing away from you, with fingers pointing upward. The left palm faces you with fingers pointing to your right. Bring the palms together.

❀ **Application** Used in the dance tradition to denote the *Kalpa* tree ("wishing tree") and mountains.

TALAMUKHA MUDRA

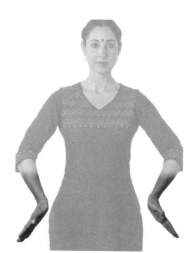

तलमुखमुद्रा

English "palms facing"

Devanagari तलमुखमुद्रा

Transliteration Talamukhamudrā

❋ **Description** *Talamukha Mudra* is a joint-hand gesture (*samyukta hasta*) noted in the *Natya Shastra* and in the *Abhinaya Darpana*. The patron deity associated with it is *Vinayaka* (*Ganesha*).

❋ **Technique** Hold the hands about 2 feet apart at hip height, with the palms facing each other at about a 45-degree angle, as if holding a *pakhawaj* (double-headed hand drum).

❋ **Application** Primarily used by performing artists to denote the following: embrace, stout, large pillar, and the lovely sounds of the drum.

Tamrachuda Mudra

ताम्रचूडमुद्रा

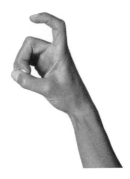

English "rooster"

Devanagari ताम्रचूडमुद्रा

Transliteration Tāmracūḍamudrā

❋ **Description** *Tamrachuda Mudra* is the twenty-seventh hand gesture of the twenty-eight single-hand mudras (*asamyukta hastas*) as described in the *Abhinaya Darpana*. According to mythology, this mudra came to exist when the three *Vedas* assumed physical form and stood before *Brahama* to make an exposition. The associated sage is *Indra*, race is *Deva*, color is mother-of-pearl, and patron deity is *Brihaspati*.

❋ **Technique** Cover the nails of the middle, ring, and little finger under the tip of the thumb. Bend the index finger like a hook.

❋ **Application** Primarily used by performing artists to create context and express emotional states or specific actions. *Viniyoga*: *Kukkuta* ("cock"); *Bhaka* ("crane"); Kaka ("crow"); *Ushtra* ("camel"); *Vathsa* ("calf"); *Lekhanam* ("writing instrument").

NOTE *Tamrachuda Mudra* is also noted in the *Natya Shastra*. However, its definition and application is identical to *Trishula Mudra* of the *Abhinaya Darpana*.

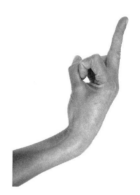

English "principle," "elemental quality," or "elemental property"

Devanagari तत्त्वमुद्रा

Transliteration Tattvamudrā

❋ **Description** *Tattva Mudra* is a single-hand gesture (*asamyukta hasta*) common to the Hindu tradition. It is used in the context of rites or rituals to signify truth, to indicate energy points on the body, traits of a deity, or to bring awareness to a given implement or sacred object.

❋ **Technique** Extend the middle finger and bend the remaining fingers toward the palm, covering the nails with the thumb.

❋ **Application** In the Hindu and yogic traditions, pointing with the index finger is considered disrespectful (since the index finger is associated with the ego). Therefore, the *Tattva Mudra* is used during ritual worship, *puja* or *yajna*, where pointing at sacred objects is called for.

❋ **Benefits** Nurtures self-respect and virtuous conduct, increases mindfulness.

TRIMUKHA MUDRA

त्रिमुखमुद्रा

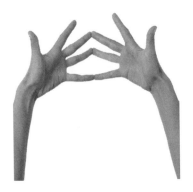

English "three faces"

Devanagari त्रिमुखमुद्रा

Transliteration Trimukhamudrā

❋ **Description** *Trimukha Mudra* is a joint-hand gesture (*samyukta hasta*) common to the yoga tradition. It is found in the *Yoga Tattva Mudra Vijnana* form, and is one of the traditional thirty-two *Gayatri Mudras*, specifically the sixth gesture in the sub-set of twenty-four mudras practiced before meditation or recitation of the *Gayatri Mantra*.

❋ **Technique** With the palms facing each other, join the tips of the middle, ring, and little fingers.

❋ **Application** In a comfortable seated position, lengthen the spine, relax the shoulders, and breathe naturally. Hold the mudra in front of the solar plexus for 5 to 45 minutes.

❋ **Benefits** Increases devotion and spiritual resolve, activates the body's self-healing power, reduces headaches, improves concentration.

त्रिपताकमुद्रा

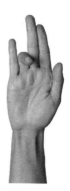

English "three parts of the flag"

Devanagari त्रिपताकमुद्रा

Transliteration Tripatākamudrā

Additional Name *Arjuna*

❋ **Description** *Tripataka Mudra* is the second hand gesture of the twenty-eight single-hand mudras (*asamyukta hastas*) as described in the *Abhinaya Darpana*. It is also noted in the *Natya Shastra* and *Abhinaya Chandrika*. According to mythology, *Indra* held his weapon, the *vajra* ("thunderbolt"), with this hand gesture. The associated sage is *Guha*, race is *Kshatriya*, color is red, and patron deity is *Shiva*.

❋ **Technique** Bend the ring finger towards the palm 90 degrees. Connect the thumb to the outer base of the index finger.

❋ **Application** Primarily used by performing artists to create context and express emotional states or specific actions. *Viniyoga*: *Makute* ("crown"); *Vrikshya-bhava* ("holy tree"); *Vajra* ("thunderbolt"); *Tat-dhara-vasava* (*Indra* "god of heaven"); *Katakikusuma* ("screw-pine flower"); *Deepam* ("oil lamp"); *Vanhi-jwala-vijrumbhana* ("rising flames"); *Kapotham* ("pigeon" or "cheeks"); *Patra-lakayam* ("to draw designs" or "write a letter"); *Bana-artha* ("arrow"); *Parivartaka* ("circular movement"); *Stri-pumsayoh-samayoge* ("union of woman and man"). Additional usages are: invocation, descent, supporting the face, bending down, recognition, disrespect, doubt, stroking the hair, marking the third eye, wearing a turban, disgust of a bad odor or harsh sound, rubbing a horse, and flight of a bird.

TRISHULA MUDRA
त्रिशूलमुद्रा

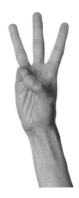

English "trident"

Devanagari त्रिशूलमुद्रा

Transliteration Triśūlamudrā

❋ **Description** *Trishula Mudra* is the twenty-eighth hand gesture of the twenty-eight single-hand mudras (*asamyukta hastas*) as described in the *Abhinaya Darpana*. It is also a ritual hand position common to the Indian Tantric and the Japanese Buddhist traditions (*Vajrayana, Mantrayana*). It is used during the rites of the *Garbhadhatu Mandala* and *Vajradhatu Mandala*.

❋ **Technique** Raise your hand with the palm facing forward. Place the pad of the thumb over the nail of the little finger. Extend and separate the index, middle, and ring fingers.

❋ **Application** In the dance and theater tradition, it is used to denote: *Bilva-patra* ("bilva leaf"); *Trithva-yukta* ("trinity"). Additional usages: the three worlds, trident, number three, wiping out tears, and the three *Vedas*. According to the Tantric Buddhist tradition, the mudra denotes a trident (spiritual weapon) and represents the extinguishing of obstacles to spiritual awakening.

❋ **Benefits** Serves as a spiritual weapon against ignorance, laziness, doubt, egoism, excessive attachment, and aversion.

NOTE In the *Natya Shastra*, this gesture is called *Tamrachuda Mudra*.

UBHAYA KARTARI MUDRA

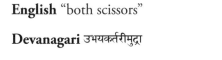

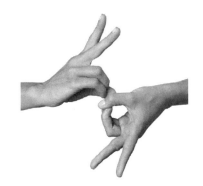

English "both scissors"

Devanagari उभयकर्तरीमुद्रा

Transliteration Ubhayakartarīmudrā

❋ **Description** *Ubhaya Kartari Mudra* is a joint-hand gesture (*samyukta hasta*) noted in the *Abhinaya Chandrika*.

❋ **Technique** Form *Kartarimukha Mudra I* (p.115) with each hand and touch the two hands at the tips of the collected thumb, ring, and little fingers.

❋ **Application** Used in Odissi Dance to denote a passionate kiss or the act of love-making between lovers.

UPADANA MUDRA

उपदानमुद्रा

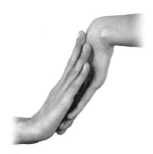

English "oblation/present"

Devanagari उपदानमुद्रा

Transliteration Upadānamudrā

* **Description** *Upadana Mudra* is a joint-hand gesture (*samyukta hasta*) common to Odissi Dance.

* **Technique** Place one hand over the other, palm to back, with the fingers pointing toward the wrists. Bend both wrists so the hands are vertical in front of your torso.

* **Application** Used to accentuate the *lasya* (feminine grace) of the dancer. Mostly used in *Pallavis* ("pure dance").

उर्णनाभमुद्रा

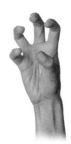

English "spider"

Devanagari उर्णनाभमुद्रा

Transliteration Urṇanābhamudrā

❋ **Description** *Urnanabha Mudra* is a single-hand gesture (*asamyukta hasta*) noted in the *Natya Shastra* and *Abhinaya Chandrika*. According to mythology, it originated from *Narasimha* (the half-man–half-lion incarnation of *Vishnu*) when he was tearing apart the chest of the demon *Hiranyakasipu*. The associated sage is *Sardulaka*, race is *Kshatriya*, color is red, and patron deity is *Adikurma*.[47]

❋ **Technique** Separate and curl all five fingers toward the palm in the shape of a claw.

❋ **Application** Used by performing artists to denote: scratching the head, theft, *Narasimha*, deer face, lion, monkey, tortoise, the *karnikara* flower, breast, fear, and blood.

USHAS MUDRA

उषस्मुद्रा

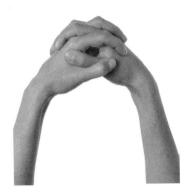

English "dawn" or "break of day"

Devanagari उषस्मुद्रा

Transliteration Uṣasmudrā

❋ **Description** *Ushas Mudra* is a joint-hand gesture (*samyukta hasta*) common to the yoga tradition. It is used to open the doorway to new opportunities and courses of action.

❋ **Technique** Clasp the hands with the left index finger on top. Bring the tips of the thumbs and index fingers toward each other, forming two open rings.

❋ **Application** This mudra may be practiced while seated, standing, or lying down. For added benefit, practice outside at sunrise facing east. Let the gentle light of the rising sun fall on your skin. Feel yourself in harmony with the fresh energy of the new day.

❋ **Benefits** Awakens body and mind in the morning hours, increases creativity and productivity, benefits the pelvis and reproductive organs, increases mental clarity and alertness, harmonizes the endocrine system.

Utsanga Mudra

उत्सङ्गमुद्रा

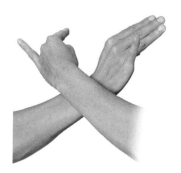

English "embrace"

Devanagari उत्सङ्गमुद्रा

Transliteration Utsaṅgamudrā

◈ **Description** *Utsanga Mudra* is the seventh hand gesture of the twenty-four joint-hand mudras (*samyukta hastas*) as described in the *Abhinaya Darpana*. It is also noted in the *Natya Shastra*. The patron deity associated with this mudra is *Gautama*.

◈ **Technique** There are several variations of this gesture. Form *Mrigashirsha* (p.158), *Arala* (p.46), or *Chatura Mudra* (p.73) with each hand. Cross the wrists with the palms facing you, and place the hands on the outer part of the upper chest.

◈ **Application** Primarily used by performing artists to create context and express emotional states or specific actions. *Viniyoga*: *Alingana* ("embrace"); *Lajayam* ("modesty" or "shyness"); *Angasa-adi-pradarshana* ("showing armlets or the body"); *Balanam-shikahana* ("nursing a baby"). It is often used to express anything to do with touch, as well as effort or anger.

NOTE The subtle specifics of this hand gesture, as well as the exact placement on the body, vary from one classical text to another.

UTTARABODHI MUDRA I

उत्तरबोधिमुद्रा

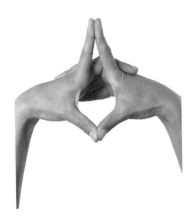

English "supreme awakening" or "perfect knowledge of the truth"

Devanagari उत्तरबोधिमुद्रा

Transliteration Uttarabodhimudrā

⁂ **Description** *Uttarabodhi Mudra I* is a joint-hand gesture (*samyukta hasta*) common to yoga tradition where it is used to connect with the source of one's inspiration.

⁂ **Technique** Interlace the fingers with the tips of the thumbs and index fingers touching. Then, press the hands together, making the opening taller and more slender.

⁂ **Application** Hold the mudra in front of the chest, with the thumbs pointing down near the end of the sternum, and index fingers pointing up. You can practice while standing, seated, or lying down. Hold for 5 to 45 minutes.

⁂ **Benefits** Soothes the nervous system, tones the large intestine (improving absorption and elimination), benefits the lungs and heart, serves as conductor of inspiration and new energy.

UTTARABODHI MUDRA II

उत्तरबोधिमुद्रा

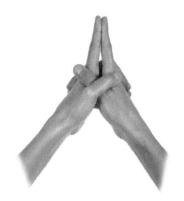

English "supreme awakening" or "perfect knowledge of the truth"

Devanagari उत्तरबोधिमुद्रा

Transliteration Uttarabodhimudrā

❊ **Description** *Uttarabodhi Mudra II* is a joint-hand gesture (*samyukta hasta*) common to the Hindu and Buddhist (*Vajrayana*) traditions, where it denotes attainment of the highest enlightenment.

❊ **Technique** Clasp the hands together with the index fingers joined and extended upward. Cross the left thumb over the right.

❊ **Application** In a comfortable seated position, lengthen the spine, relax the shoulders and chest, and breathe naturally. Rest the mudra against the sternum, with the index fingers pointing upward. Feel the top of your head extending upward and your tailbone rooting to the center of the Earth. Feel a sense of openness in body and mind. Relax in stillness and hold for 5 to 45 minutes.

❊ **Benefits** Increases mental clarity, strengthens willpower, clears the central channel (*sushumna nadi*), makes the body feel light and rooted at the same time, works like a lightning rod to attract inspiration and insight.

VAIRAGYA MUDRA

वैराग्यमुद्रा

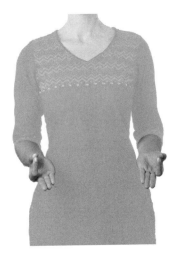

English "conscious detachment" or "absence of worldly desires"

Devanagari वैराग्यमुद्रा

Transliteration Vairāgyamudrā

Additional Name *Veragya*

❋ **Description** *Vairagya Mudra* is a joint-hand gesture (*samyukta hasta*) common to the yoga tradition. It is found in the *Yoga Tattva Mudra Vijnana* form, and is one of the traditional thirty-two *Gayatri Mudras*, specifically the third gesture in the sub-set of eight mudras practiced after meditation or recitation of the *Gayatri Mantra*.

❋ **Technique** Join the tips of the thumbs and index fingers of each hand. Place the hands lightly on the thighs, palms facing upward.

❋ **Application** In a comfortable seated position, lengthen the spine, relax the shoulders and belly, and breathe naturally. Focus inward, feeling the hands like the two sides of a scale. Notice the feeling in your body and mind as you adjust your posture subtly to balance this scale. Hold for 5 to 45 minutes.

❋ **Benefits** Improves memory, imparts a sense of balance and equanimity, increases mental and emotional flexibility, improves one's ability to flow with changing circumstances, serves as an energy seal during meditation.

VAJRA MUDRA

वज्रमुद्रा

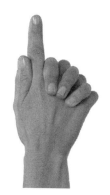

English "thunderbolt" or "adamantine"

Devanagari वज्रमुद्रा

Transliteration Vajramudrā

* **Description** *Vajra Mudra* is a joint-hand gesture (*samyukta hasta*) common to the yoga tradition, where it is used to focus the mind and direct *prana* (vital energy).

* **Technique** Clasp the hands with the index fingers extended. Lightly press the sides of the thumbs together, touching the pads to the outsides of the index fingers.

* **Application** *Vajra Mudra* may be practiced standing, seated, or lying down. Hold the mudra in front of the chest. Relax the shoulders and breathe naturally. Hold for 5 to 45 minutes.

* **Benefits** Aligns and opens the central channel (*sushumna nadi*), directs energy upward to the higher centers in the body, improves concentration, and strengthens willpower.

NOTE One of the most effective ways to practice this mudra is to kneel on the floor in *Vajrasana* (thunderbolt pose), holding the mudra overhead, with the index fingers pointing skyward.

VAJRAPRADANA MUDRA

वज्रप्रदानमुद्रा

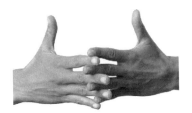

English "unswerving trust" or "unshakable confidence"

Devanagari वज्रप्रदानमुद्रा

Transliteration Vajrapradānamudrā

Additional Name *Vajrashraddha*

* **Description** *Vajrapradana Mudra* is a joint-hand gesture (*samyukta hasta*) common to the yoga tradition where it is used to show unshakable trust in the *Dharma*.

* **Technique** Interlace the fingers at the top knuckle. The thumbs remain extended upward.

* **Application** In a comfortable seated position, lengthen the spine, relax the shoulders and belly, and breathe naturally. Focus inward, feeling confidence arise in your chosen path or spiritual practice. Hold for 5 to 45 minutes.

* **Benefits** Increases spiritual confidence, promotes humility, increases one's commitment to spiritual life.

NOTE This mudra can be used during prayer, especially while expressing desire for spiritual guidance or assistance on the path of spiritual cultivation.

वलितमुद्रा

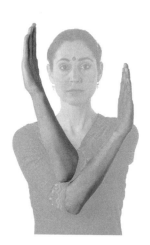

English "bent around" or "cooperation"

Devanagari वलितमुद्रा

Transliteration Valitamudrā

※ **Description** *Valita Mudra* is a joint-hand dance gesture (*samyukta hasta*) noted in the *Natya Shastra*. *Valita Mudra* creatively frames the face to accentuate theatrical expressions.

※ **Technique** Cross the arms at the elbows. Maintain flat palms with the fingers extended and collected. Palms face to the sides as they frame the face.

※ **Application** Used as an esthetically pleasing formation in *Nritta* ("pure dance").

Varada Mudra

वरदमुद्रा

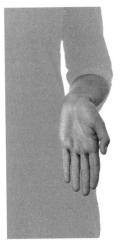

English "wish fulfilling"

Devanagari वरदमुद्रा

Transliteration Varadamudrā

◈ **Description** *Varada Mudra* is a single-hand gesture (*asamyukta hasta*) common to the Hindu and Buddhist traditions. It signifies offering, welcome, charity, giving, compassion, and sincerity.

◈ **Technique** With the palm facing forward and the fingers collected, turn the tips of the fingers to point toward the ground.

◈ **Application** Usually used in the context of rites or rituals, such as an initiation ceremony or taking of vows. It is most commonly seen in iconographic depictions (painting and sculpture) of a deity, sage, or saint, where it is generally held with the left hand, while another gesture—often *Abhaya Mudra*—is formed with the right.

◈ **Benefits** The benefit of *Varada Mudra* is traditionally associated with the onlooker witnessing the mudra instead of the person performing it. In this case, the mudra becomes like a *yantra* or *mandala*, and can be used as an object of contemplation

NOTE In the dance tradition, the combination of *Varada* and *Abhaya Mudra* is often used to depict *Parvati* or any of the other various emanations of the goddess.

VARAHA MUDRA I

वराहमुद्रा

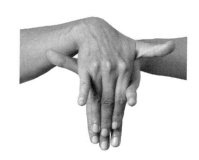

English "boar"

Devanagari वराहमुद्रा

Transliteration Varāhamudrā

* **Description** *Varaha Mudra I* is the nineteenth hand gesture of the twenty-four joint-hand mudras (*samyukta hastas*) as described in the *Abhinaya Darpana*.

* **Technique** Place the right palm over the back of the left hand. Bend the index, middle, and ring fingers at the base joint, maintaining extended and collected fingers. Stretch the little fingers directly forward to represent the tusks of the boar, and extend your thumbs sideways to represent the ears of the boar.

* **Application** Used by performing artists to denote a boar. *Varaha is* known in the Hindu tradition as the third incarnation ("*avatara*") of *Vishnu*. To indicate the movement of the boar, undulate the wrists in an up-and-down motion.

VARAHA MUDRA II

वराहमुद्रा

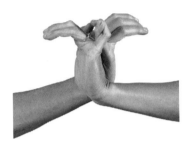

English "boar"

Devanagari वराहमुद्रा

Transliteration Varāhamudrā

- ❁ **Description** *Varaha Mudra II* is a less common variation of the nineteenth hand gesture of the twenty-four joint-hand mudras (*samyukta hastas*) as described in the *Abhinaya Darpana*.

- ❁ **Technique** Bring the backs of the hands together with fingers pointing upward. Interlock the thumbs and little fingers. Curve the index, middle, and little fingers of each hand.

- ❁ **Application** Used by performing artists to denote a wild boar.

VARAHA MUDRA III

वराहमुद्रा

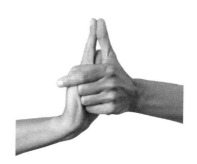

English "boar"

Devanagari वराहमुद्रा

Transliteration Varāhamudrā

* **Description** *Varaha Mudra III* is a joint-hand gesture (*samyukta hasta*) common to the yoga tradition. It is found in the *Yoga Tattva Mudra Vijnana* form, and is one of the traditional thirty-two *Gayatri Mudras*, specifically the twentieth gesture in the sub-set of twenty-four mudras practiced before meditation or recitation of the *Gayatri Mantra*.

* **Technique** Hold the left hand with the palm facing you. Curl the middle, ring, and little fingers toward the palm with the index finger pointing to the right and the thumb extended upward. With the right hand, clasp the curled fingers of the left. Connect the right index finger to the left thumb. The left index finger rests on the outside of the right little finger.

* **Application** In a comfortable seated position, hold the mudra in front of the chest. Lengthen the spine, relax the shoulders and belly, and breathe naturally. Hold for 5 to 45 minutes.

* **Benefits** Activates the body's self-healing power, balances the immune system, increases courage and resourcefulness.

Vardhamana Mudra

वर्धमानमुद्रा

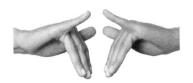

English "increasing"

Devanagari वर्धमानमुद्रा

Transliteration Vardhamānamudrā

❊ **Description** *Vardhamana Mudra* is a joint-hand gesture (*samyukta hasta*) noted in the *Abhinaya Darpana* and *Natya Shastra*. The patron deity associated is *Vasuki*.[48]

❊ **Technique** Form *Hamsapaksha Mudra* (p.95) with each hand, fingers pointing downward, hands separated in front of your body.

❊ **Application** Indicates the opening of things such as curtains, as well as the violent act of tearing a demon's chest apart by a fierce deity or protector.[49] The dynamic action requires the turning of the palms upward.

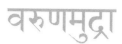

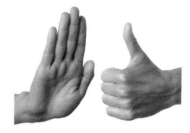

English "of the sea" or "god of the sea"

Devanagari वरुणमुद्रा

Transliteration Varuṇamudrā

❋ **Description** *Varuna Mudra I* is a joint-hand gesture (*samyukta hasta*) used by performing artists. It is found in the traditional set of sixteen *Deva Hastas*, denoting Hindu gods and goddesses as described in the *Abhinaya Darpana*. It indicates the form and character of the Hindu deity *Varuna*.

❋ **Technique** Assume *Shikhara Mudra* (p.225) with your left hand and *Pataka Mudra* (p.186) with your right hand. Hold both hands in front of your chest.

❋ **Application** It is used to indicate *Varuna*, the god of the oceans, water, and sky ("celestial ocean").

NOTE There are several combinations of mudras used to express the various traits and emblems of *Varuna Deva*. The one indicated here appears to be the most common.

VARUNA MUDRA II

वरुणमुद्रा

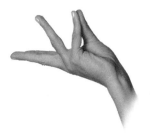

English "of the sea" or "god of the sea"

Devanagari वरुणमुद्रा

Transliteration Varuṇamudrā

- **Description** *Varuna Mudra II* is single-hand gesture (*asamyukta hasta*) common to the yoga tradition. It is used in the *Yoga Tattva Mudra Vijnana* form to access the intelligence of the Water Element, and to increase the abundance of love, passion, and wholesome sexual expression.

- **Technique** Lightly join the tips of the thumb and little finger, leaving the remaining fingers relaxed.

- **Application** In a comfortable seated position, form the mudra with each hand and rest the hands on the thighs, palms facing up. With gratitude, connect with the spirit of water, feeling your body and mind become pure and fresh, like a cool mountain stream. Hold for 5 to 45 minutes.

- **Benefits** Cooling and calming, cures excessive thirst, reduces wrinkles and dryness of the skin, increases overall suppleness of the body, benefits the tendons, ligaments, and muscles, strengthens kidneys and bladder, nourishes and cleanses the blood and lymph, improves memory, tones the sexual organs and assists healing from trauma related to sexual abuse or shame around sexuality, awakens inner joy and vitality, enhances overall physical beauty.

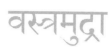

वस्त्रमुद्रा

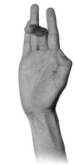

English "cloth" or "clothing"

Devanagari वस्त्रमुद्रा

Transliteration Vastramudrā

❀ **Description** *Vastra Mudra* is a single-hand gesture (*asamyukta hasta*) noted in the *Abhinaya Chandrika*. It is common to the Odissi Dance tradition.

❀ **Technique** With the palm facing forward and the fingers extended, bend the middle finger 90 degrees at the second joint.

❀ **Application** Used to denote items of clothing.

Vayu Mudra I

वायुमुद्रा

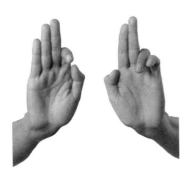

English "wind" or "air"

Devanagari वायुमुद्रा

Transliteration Vāyumudrā

Additional names *Vata, Pavana, Prana*

* **Description** *Vayu Mudra I* is a joint-hand gesture (*samyukta hasta*) used by performing artists. It is found in the traditional set of sixteen *Deva Hastas*, denoting Hindu gods and goddesses as described in the *Abhinaya Darpana*. It indicates the form and character of the Hindu deity *Vayu*.

* **Technique** Form *Ardhapataka Mudra* (p.50) with your left hand and *Arala Mudra* (p.46) with your right. Hold both hands in front of your chest.

* **Application** Used to indicate *Vayu*, the god of air and wind.

Note There are several combinations of mudras used to express the various traits and emblems of *Vayu Deva*. The one indicated here appears to be the most common.

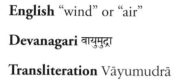

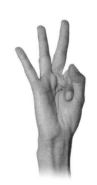

English "wind" or "air"

Devanagari वायुमुद्रा

Transliteration Vāyumudrā

    Description *Vayu Mudra II* is a single-hand gesture (*asamyukta hasta*) common to the yoga tradition. It is found in the *Yoga Tattva Mudra Vijnana* form where it is used to treat complications related to the Air Element by controlling and balancing *Vata Dosha* (see Appendix A).

    Technique Touch the tip of the index finger to the base of the thumb, with the thumb covering the index finger. Keep the other three fingers extended and relaxed.

    Application *Vayu Mudra* may be used anytime in any position: walking, standing, sitting, or lying down. It is more effective to hold the mudra with each hand. For treatment of health conditions, it is ideal to practice 2 to 3 sessions per day of 10 to 45 minutes. Once the desired effects have been attained, discontinue regular practice of *Vayu Mudra* and continue a daily practice of *Prana Mudra*, *Varuna Mudra* and/or *Prithivi Mudra*.

    Benefits Reduces gas, bloating, and belching, treats diseases such as polio, gout, arthritis, sciatica, and muscular trembling (as is common in Parkinson's disease).

NOTE *Vayu Mudra* yields improved results when practiced after *Prana Mudra* in a given session.

Vayu Mudra III

वायुमुद्रा

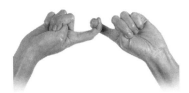

English "wind" or "air"

Devanagari वायुमुद्रा

Transliteration Vāyumudrā

❋ **Description** *Vayu Mudra III* is a joint-hand gesture (*samyukta hasta*) common to the Buddhist *Vajrayana* tradition. It is a Tantric mudra held by priests during performance of the *Garbhadhatu Mandala* ("Womb Realm") and the *Vajradhatu Mandala* ("Diamond Realm") rites, where it symbolizes the auspicious wind that scatters delusion and clears obstacles.

❋ **Technique** Touch the tip of the thumb to the base of the ring finger, and close the middle, ring, and little finger over the thumb. Hook the two index fingers at the first knuckle.

❋ **Application** In a comfortable seated position, lengthen the spine, relax the shoulders and belly, and breathe naturally. Hold for 5 to 45 minutes.

❋ **Benefits** Removes obstacles on the spiritual path, such as laziness, doubt, ignorance, egoism, excessive craving and aversion, and so on.

Venu Mudra

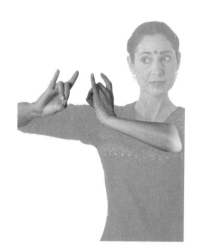

वेणुमुद्रा

English "flute"

Devanagari वेणुमुद्रा

Transliteration Veṇumudrā

❋ **Description** *Venu Mudra* is common to the Odissi Dance tradition where it is used to express the character of *Krishna*. It can be performed with one or two hands.

❋ **Technique** With each hand, join the tips of the middle and ring fingers with the tip of the thumb, forming a circle. Keep the little finger and index finger extended upward and slightly curved. Hold the hands to the right side of the mouth, as if playing a flute.

❋ **Application** Used exclusively to depict *Krishna*, as the *venu* flute is his most common icon.

Vighneshvara Mudra

विघ्नेश्वरमुद्रा

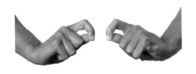

English "remover of obstacles"

Devanagari विघ्नेश्वरमुद्रा

Transliteration Vighneśvaramudrā

Additional names *Ganesha, Ganapati, Gajanana, Vighnarat, Vinayaka*

* **Description** *Vighneshvara Mudra* is a joint-hand gesture (*samyukta hasta*) used by performing artists. It is found in the traditional set of sixteen *Deva Hastas,* denoting Hindu gods and goddesses as described in the *Abhinaya Darpana.* It indicates the form and character of the Hindu deity *Ganesha.*

* **Technique** Form *Kapittha Mudra* (p.106) with each hand, held about 6 inches in front of the hips.

* **Application** Used to indicate *Ganesha,* the remover of obstacles.

NOTE There are several combinations of mudras used to express the various traits and emblems of *Ganesha Deva.* The one indicated here appears to be the most common.

VISHNU MUDRA I

विष्णुमुद्रा

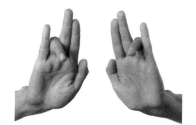

English "god of preservation"

Devanagari विष्णुमुद्रा

Transliteration Viṣṇumudrā

※ **Description** *Vishnu Mudra I* is a joint-hand gesture (*samyukta hasta*) used by performing artists. It is found in the traditional set of sixteen *Deva Hastas*, denoting Hindu gods and goddesses as described in the *Abhinaya Darpana*. It indicates the form and character of the Hindu deity *Vishnu*.

※ **Technique** Assume *Tripataka Mudra* (p.253) with each hand. Stand with your feet hip width apart. Hold the hands in front of the shoulders with the elbows at shoulder height, bending the wrists so your palms face away from you.

※ **Application** Used to indicate *Vishnu*, who is worshipped as the supreme god in the *Vaishnava* tradition of Hinduism.

NOTE There are several combinations of mudras used to express the various traits and emblems of *Vishnu Deva*. The one indicated here appears to be the most common. *Vishnu* is also represented through the mudras of the ten incarnations (*Dashavatara*). See Appendix C.

VISHNU MUDRA II
विष्णुमुद्रा

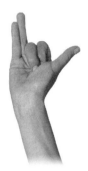

English "god of preservation"

Devanagari विष्णुमुद्रा

Transliteration Viṣṇumudrā

* **Description** *Vishnu Mudra II* is a single-hand gesture (*asamyukta hasta*) common to the yoga tradition. It is used primarily during the practice of *pranayama* (breathing exercises) to control the left and right nostrils during techniques such as *Nadi Shodhana Pranayama.*[50]

* **Technique** Raise the right hand and fold the index and middle fingers into the palm. Extend the thumb, ring, and little fingers.

* **Application** Use *Vishnu Mudra* to control the volume of air passing through the nostrils during breathing exercises.[51]

* **Benefits** Provides a comfortable and elegant way to employ the delicate pressure required to control the opening and closing of the nostrils during the practice of *pranayama*.

NOTE In the dance tradition, the same hand gesture is used to denote the *amalaka* tree. It is known as *Samyama Nayaka Mudra* in the *Abhinaya Darpana*.

विशुद्धचक्रमुद्रा

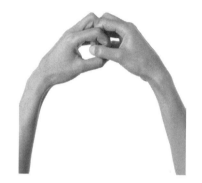

English "purified"

Devanagari विशुद्धचक्रमुद्रा

Transliteration Viśuddhacakramudrā

※ **Description** *Vishuddha Chakra Mudra* is a joint-hand gesture (*samyukta hasta*) used in Tantric Yoga and Japanese martial arts to open the *Vishuddha Chakra* (the throat energy center) and improve communication.

※ **Technique** Interlace the fingers with the tips pointing toward the palm. Join the tips of the index fingers and thumbs, forming two interlocking rings.

※ **Application** In a comfortable seated position, hold the mudra in front of the throat. Place the tip of the tongue on the upper palate, and relax the shoulders and chest. Bring your attention to the spacious feeling inside the throat and neck. Settle into stillness and listen to the inner silence. Hold for 5 to 45 minutes.

※ **Benefits** Improves the health of the thyroid and parathyroid glands, benefits the voice, reduces tension in the neck, improves communication with self and others, increases sensitivity to the thoughts and feelings of others.

VISTARA MUDRA
विस्तरमुद्रा

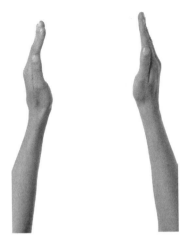

English "expansion"

Devanagari विस्तरमुद्रा

Transliteration Vistaramudrā

Additional Name *Vistritam*

❋ **Description** *Vistara Mudra* is a joint-hand gesture (*samykta hasta*) common to the yoga tradition. It is found in the *Yoga Tattva Mudra Vijnana* form, and is one of the traditional thirty-two *Gayatri Mudras*, specifically the fourth gesture in the sub-set of twenty-four mudras practiced before meditation or recitation of the *Gayatri Mantra*.

❋ **Technique** Raise the hands in front of the belly, palms facing the midline, about 10 inches apart.

❋ **Application** In a comfortable seated position, lengthen the spine and relax the belly. Adjust your breathing to be slow and deep, feeling the belly expand with the inhalation and contract with the exhalation. With the mudra in front of your abdomen, feel a sense of thickness between your hands. Allow the hands to move ever so slightly apart as you inhale, and back toward each other as you exhale. Practice this way for 5 to 20 minutes.

❋ **Benefits** Reduces arthritic pain in the hands, increases sensitivity to energy, improves blood circulation, awakens the body's self-healing capacity, improves healing abilities.

NOTE It is ideal to practice *Vistara Mudra* after you develop sensitivity to the feeling of energy through the practice of *Vitita Mudra*.

VITITA MUDRA
विtitमुद्रा

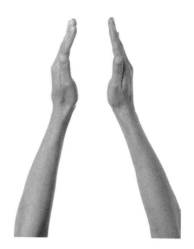

English "bloom"

Devanagari विtitमुद्रा

Transliteration Vititamudrā

⁕ **Description** *Vitita Mudra* is a joint-hand gesture (*samyukta hasta*) common to the yoga tradition. It is found in the *Yoga Tattva Mudra Vijnana* form, and is one of the traditional thirty-two *Gayatri Mudras*, specifically the third gesture in the sub-set of twenty-four mudras practiced before meditation or recitation of the *Gayatri Mantra*.

⁕ **Technique** Raise the hands in front of the belly, palms facing the midline, about 3 inches apart.

⁕ **Application** In a comfortable seated position, lengthen the spine and relax the shoulders, chest, and belly. Adjust your breathing to be slow, smooth, deep, and even. Feel the belly expand with the inhalation and contract with the exhalation. With the mudra held in front of your abdomen, feel a sense of thickness between your hands. Allow the hands to move ever so slightly apart as you inhale, and back together as you exhale. Practice this way for 5 to 20 minutes.

⁕ **Benefits** Reduces arthritic pain in the hands, increases sensitivity to energy, improves blood circulation, activates the body's self-healing power, strengthens healing abilities.

VYANA MUDRA

व्यानमुद्रा

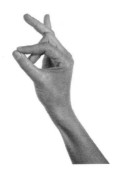

English "all-pervading," "outward flowing," or "integrated"

Devanagari व्यानमुद्रा

Transliteration Vyānamudrā

⁂ **Description** *Vyana Mudra* is a single-hand gesture (*asamyukta hasta*) common to the yoga tradition. It is found in the *Yoga Tattva Mudra Vijnana* form where it is used primarily to lower blood pressure.

⁂ **Technique** Join the tips of the thumb and index finger. Touch the tip of the middle finger to the middle line of the thumb. Extend the ring and little fingers upward.

⁂ **Application** In a comfortable seated position, form the mudra with each hand and place the hands in the lap, palms up. Lengthen the spine, relax the shoulders and belly, and breathe naturally. Hold for 5 to 45 minutes.

⁂ **Benefits** Regulates the blood pressure, purifies the blood, decreases restlessness and insomnia, reduces redness and burning of the eyes.

Vyapak Anjali Mudra

व्यापकाञ्जलिमुद्रा

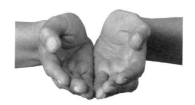

English "all-pervading offerings"

Devanagari व्यापकाञ्जलिमुद्रा

Transliteration Vyāpakāñjalimudrā

* **Description** *Vyapak Anjali Mudra* is a joint-hand gesture (*samyukta hasta*) common to the yoga tradition. It is found in the *Yoga Tattva Mudra Vijnana* form, and is one of the traditional thirty-two *Gayatri Mudras*, specifically the eleventh gesture in the sub-set of twenty-four mudras practiced before meditation or recitation of the *Gayatri Mantra*.

* **Technique** With the palms facing upward, curve the hands slightly and join the outer edges of the little fingers to create a basket-like shape in front of the heart center.

* **Application** In a comfortable seated position, lengthen the spine and relax the shoulders. Adjust your breathing to be slow and deep. With the mudra held in front of your heart, visualize filling your hands with all the love, compassion, and good will you can imagine. With utmost sincerity, make an offering of these virtues to benefit all beings in limitless time and space. See a connection from your heart to each individual being. Continue making offerings this way for 5 to 45 minutes (or until tears of compassion run down your cheeks).

* **Benefits** Lifts depression and cures excessive self-consciousness and even self-hatred, ignites the heart of true compassion for self and others, increases devotion and commitment to honestly living a spiritual life.

NOTE In the version shown here, the hands are slightly cupped. However, the mudra is often seen practiced with the hands in a more flat position, resembling an offering platter.

YAMA MUDRA

यममुद्रा

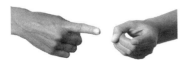

English "god of death"

Devanagari यममुद्रा

Transliteration Yamamudrā

Additional Name *Yamaraja*

❋ **Description** *Yama Mudra* is a joint-hand gesture (*samyukta hasta*) used by performing artists. It is found in the traditional set of sixteen *Deva Hastas*, denoting Hindu gods and goddesses as described in the *Abhinaya Darpana*. It indicates the form and character of the Hindu deity *Yama*.

❋ **Technique** Form *Tamrachuda Mudra* (p.250) with your left hand and *Suchi Mudra* (p.240) with your right hand. Hold the left hand in front of your waist, slightly to your left. Point to the left hand with the right index finger.

❋ **Application** It is used to indicate *Yama*, the Hindu god of death. The left hand simulates a hook, which denotes the way death "hooks" his victims when they are ready to submit themselves to the inevitable.

NOTE There are several combinations of mudras used to express the various traits and emblems of *Yama Deva*. The one indicated here appears to be the most common.

यमपाशमुद्रा

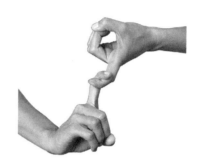

English "noose of death"

Devanagari यमपाशमुद्रा

Transliteration Yamapāśamudrā

❋ **Description** *Yampasha Mudra* is a joint-hand gesture (*samyukta hasta*) common to the yoga tradition. It is found in the *Yoga Tattva Mudra Vijnana* form, and is one of the traditional thirty-two *Gayatri Mudras*, specifically the thirteenth gesture in the sub-set of twenty-four mudras practiced before meditation or recitation of the *Gayatri Mantra*.

❋ **Technique** On each hand, extend the index fingers and join the remaining fingers together with the thumb. Hook the index fingers, with the left hand facing up and the right hand facing down.

❋ **Application** In a comfortable seated position, lengthen the spine and relax the shoulders, chest, and belly. Adjust your breathing to be slow, smooth, and even. Hold the mudra in front of your heart for 5 to 20 minutes.

❋ **Benefits** Opens the airways, strengthens the lungs and large intestine, stimulates the immune system, evokes the spiritual insight of the interdependent nature of all phenomena (death creates life, life creates death).

Yoni Mudra I
योनिमुद्रा

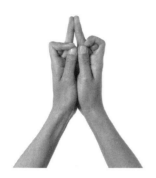

English "vulva" or "origin"

Devanagari योनिमुद्रा

Transliteration Yonimudrā

BACK

❋ **Description** *Yoni Mudra I* is an intricate joint-hand gesture (*samyukta hasta*) common to the yoga tradition. It is found in the *Yoga Tattva Mudra Vijnana* form, and is one of the traditional thirty-two *Gayatri Mudras*, specifically the fourth gesture in the sub-set of eight mudras practiced after meditation or recitation of the *Gayatri Mantra*.

❋ **Technique** Join the palms together in front of the chest. Cross the ring fingers and open the hand like a book. Place the right ring finger on top of the left middle finger. Place the left ring finger on top of the right middle finger. Hook the tip of the right ring finger with the left index, and hook the tip of the left ring finger with the right index. Close the hands slowly, bringing the pads of the middle fingers together. The little fingers are crossed in back and the thumbs are parallel.

❋ **Application** In a comfortable seated position, hold the mudra in front of the heart or pelvis. Place the tip of the tongue on the upper palate, and relax the shoulders and chest. Bring your attention to the spacious feeling inside the heart and watery feeling inside the pelvis. Settle into stillness and, without judging or interfering, simply be receptive to whatever arises. Hold for 5 to 45 minutes.

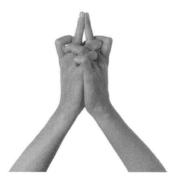

FRONT

Benefits Improves the health of the sexual organs, invites a healthy sense of sacredness around sexuality, increases receptivity, fluidity, and emotional sensitivity, serves as a gateway to embrace what we can't understand (mystery), creates a physical mandala to worship the Divine Feminine.

NOTE The effects of practicing *Yoni Mudra* can be enhanced by chanting traditional mantras associated with *Shakti* or *Devi*, or by singing *bhajans* (spiritual songs) dedicated to the Divine Mother or any of the many aspects of the goddess.

Yoni Mudra II
योनिमुद्रा

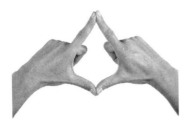

English "vulva" or "origin"

Devanagari योनिमुद्रा

Transliteration Yonimudrā

⁂ **Description** *Yoni Mudra II* is a joint-hand gesture (*samyukta hasta*) common to the Hindu and Buddhist *Vajrayana* traditions. It is a Tantric mudra usually employed by priests or devotees during performance of sacred rites or rituals.

⁂ **Technique** Extend the index fingers and thumbs of each hand, folding the remaining fingers into the palm. Join the tips of the extended fingers, forming a triangular shape.

⁂ **Application** There are two main applications of this mudra: (1) hold the gesture in front of the heart with the index fingers pointing upward; (2) hold the mudra in front of the pelvis with the index fingers pointing downward. Ideally, the upward (masculine) and downward (feminine) versions of the mudra are practiced together in a single session. Start by practicing 5 minutes in each position, and build up time, as you feel ready. So long as your breathing remains calm and natural, and your shoulders and chest stay relaxed, you may practice for as long as you like.

⁂ **Benefits** Harmonizes the sexual and spiritual energies within the body, creates a connection between the heart (love) and the sexual glands (creative energy).

योनिमुद्रा

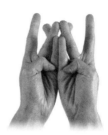

English "vulva" or "origin"

Devanagari योनिमुद्रा

Transliteration Yonimudrā

- **Description** *Yoni Mudra III* is a joint-hand gesture (*samyukta hasta*) common to the yoga tradition. It is found in the *Yoga Tattva Mudra Vijnana* form, and is one of the traditional thirty-two *Gayatri Mudras*, specifically the fourth gesture in the sub-set of eight mudras practiced after meditation or recitation of the *Gayatri Mantra*.

- **Technique** Turn the palms upward and join the hands at the outer edges. Cross the right ring finger over the left, join the tips of the middle fingers, and connect the outer edges of the little fingers. Touch the tips of the thumbs to the bases of the little fingers.

- **Application** In a comfortable seated position, hold the mudra in front of the heart. Place the tip of the tongue on the upper palate, and relax the shoulders and chest. Bring your attention to the spacious feeling inside the heart and watery feeling inside the pelvis. Settle into stillness and, without judging or interfering, simply be receptive to whatever arises. Hold for 5 to 45 minutes.

- **Benefits** Improves the health of the kidneys and bladder, benefits the sexual glands (testes in men, ovaries in women), reduces dryness in the body, increases the luster of the skin and hair, strengthens connection with the principal of the Divine Feminine, increases devotion and loving kindness.

NOTE Although they are different in appearance, *Yoni Mudra III* and *Yoni Mudra I* are considered to have similar healing properties and spiritual significance, and are used interchangeably in different traditions of yoga.

APPENDIX A

Energy Anatomy

The Seven Chakras of Indian Tantric Yoga

1. **Muladhara Chakra**—*mula* ("base" or "root"), *adhara* ("support")

   Location: Perineum, below genitals, above anus, base of spine

   Element: Earth

   Number of Petals: 4

   Elemental Color: Shining yellow[1]

   Ruling Planet: Mars

   Governs: Feet, legs, anus, and elimination

   Positive Attributes: Stability, loyalty

   Negative Attributes: Stubbornness, heavy mindedness

2. **Svadhishthana Chakra**—*sva* ("self"), *adhisthana* ("dwelling place")

   Location: Genital region

   Element: Water

   Number of Petals: 6

   Elemental Color: Light blue

   Ruling Planet: Mercury

   Governs: Reproductive system, power to create

   Positive Attributes: Flexibility, openness, intuitiveness

   Negative Attributes: Ungrounded-ness, unconscious leakage of sexual energy

3. **Manipura Chakra**—*mani* ("jewel"), *pura* ("filled with" or "city")

    Location: Behind navel, toward spine

    Element: Fire

    Number of Petals: 10

    Elemental Color: Sunrise red

    Ruling Planet: Sun

    Governs: Digestion, assimilation

    Positive Attributes: Zest for life, vitality, self-control

    Negative Attributes: Ruthlessness, abuse of power, self-abuse

4. **Anahata Chakra**—("un-struck sound")

    Location: Heart region of the spine

    Element: Air

    Number of Petals: 12

    Elemental Color: Smoky grey

    Ruling Planet: Venus

    Governs: Heart, diaphragm, lungs, arms, and hands

    Positive Attributes: Devotion, love, compassion

    Negative Attributes: Attachment, rampant emotions, hate

5. **Vishudha Chakra**—("pure")

    Location: Throat area

    Element: Ether/Space

    Number of Petals: 16

    Elemental Color: White (like the full moon)

    Ruling Planet: Jupiter

    Governs: Speech, thyroid, parathyroid

    Positive Attributes: Expansiveness, silence, deep calm

    Negative Attributes: Spacey-ness, boredom, restlessness

6. **Ajna Chakra**—("enhanced knowledge")

   Location: Point between eyebrows, base of skull

   Element: Mind

   Number of Petals: 2

   Elemental Color: Pure white

   Ruling Planet: Saturn

   Governs: Intellect, seat of enlightenment

   Positive Attributes: Alignment, radiant joy, wisdom

   Negative Attributes: Overly intellectual, coldly rational

7. **Sahasrara Chakra**—("thousand petalled")

   Location: Above the top of the head

   Element: None

   Number of Petals: Infinite

   Elemental Color: Clear light, colorless

   Ruling Planet: None

   Governs: Doorway to non-duality

   Attributes: Non-duality, beyond positive/negative, infinite

The Five Vayus

Through thousands of years of research into the functioning of the human body-mind, ancient yogis discovered that *prana* flows in distinct ways in certain areas of the body. They likened these patterns to the way currents and eddies function in a moving river, and found these unique energies play important roles in the functioning of related tissues and organs. Their findings are summarized in what is called the theory of the Five Winds (*Pancha Vayu*).

1. *Apana Vayu* ("downward wind")—resides in the pelvis and legs, governs the organs of elimination and reproduction.

2. *Prana Vayu* ("vital wind")—resides in the chest region (from the throat to the navel), governs the heart and lungs and serves to "fill" all the other *vayus* with vigor.

3. *Samana Vayu* ("stable wind")—resides in the abdomen, governs the organs of digestion and assimilation.

4. *Udana Vayu* ("rising wind")—resides in the head and neck, governs speech, swallowing, the eyes, brain, and hair.

5. *Vyana Vayu* ("pervading wind")—the roaming *vayu*; located everywhere in the body, this *vayu* serves to coalesce and harmonize the other four into a cohesive whole.

Five Fingers and Five Elements

Finger (English)	Finger (Sanskrit)	Element (English)	Element (Sanskrit)
Thumb	*Angushtha*	Fire	*Agni*
Index	*Tarjani*	Air	*Vayu*
Middle	*Madhya*	Ether/Space	*Akasha*
Ring	*Anamika*	Earth	*Prithivi*
Little	*Kanishthika*	Water	*Apas*

The Three Doshas

Dosha literally means ("blemish") or ("tendency toward imbalance"). The human experience is colored by the dance of three *doshas*: *Vata, Pitta, and Kapha*. The interplay of these three powers largely determines the health of the body-mind, the rate of aging, and the susceptibility to disease. In each individual, one of the three *doshas* predominates and determines the basic constitution, or body-mind "type."

1. *Vata* (Air + Ether/Space)—*Vata* literally means ("wind"). It is composed of air in movement and ether (space) in substance. *Vata* is the motivating force behind the other two *doshas*. It exists as the empty spaces in the body: joints, hollow organs, the bone cavities of the hips and low back. More subtly, *Vata* moves in the inner space of mind. Disturbed *Vata* produces: mental nervousness, digestive disorders (gas), low energy, drying and weakening of body tissues. Since *Vata* is the origin of the other two *doshas*, its health depends on the amount of *Pitta* and *Kapha* present to balance and stabilize it. Unstabilized *Vata* moves so much it burns itself out.

2. *Pitta* (Fire + Water)—*Pitta* literally means ("cooking") or ("digesting power"). Since fire cannot exist directly in the body, *Pitta* is the fire held in the water and oil of the cells. It is the heat of transformation and digestion held in the body's tissues. More subtly, it is the force that allows for "digestion" and "assimilation" of life's experiences to create meaning and understanding. Imbalanced *Pitta* can manifest as excess toxic build-up, infection, inflammation, acid, and irritability. The health of *Pitta* depends on *Vata* for smooth movement and *Kapha* for grounding.

3. *Kapha* (Water + Earth)—*Kapha* literally means ("what makes things stick together"). *Kapha* is the power of cohesion. *Kapha* is water held in the medium of earth. In the body, *Kapha's* root is the plasma, and its presence can be noted in the mucous linings, the heavy oily substances of the body. Imbalanced *Kapha* can manifest as excess mucus, fat, sluggishness, dull mind, swollen glands, or feeling stuck in life. *Kapha* depends on *Vata* for its stimulus to move, and *Pitta* to keep it warm enough to move at all. Simply put, if *Kapha* doesn't move, it stagnates and develops into disease.

Each person has a unique blend of the three *doshas*. The presence of each dosha in varying amounts makes up their signature constitution. For example, a person with a dominance of *Pitta* as well as a high level of *Vata* would be considered a *Pitta Vata* type. There is no one type that is better or more desirable; each has its benefits and difficulties. What is paramount to take from the theory of *doshas*, and its relationship to mudras, is that we can use the methods of yoga and Ayurveda to skillfully bring our unique constitution into balance to sustain a life of radiant health and happiness.

APPENDIX B

The Gayatri Mudras

The thirty-two *Gayatri Mudras* listed below are a traditional set of Vedic hand gestures corresponding to the practice of *Gayatri Japa* (recitation of the *Gayatri Mantra*). For many ardent devotees of the Vedic tradition, performance of *Gayatri sadhana* ("devoted practice") is done three times per day: sunrise, noon, and sunset. Slow, rhythmic execution of the *mudras*, along with the chanting of the mantra, is said to completely balance body and mind, impart good health and longevity, and illuminate the spirit of the *sadhaka* (practitioner). The *Gayatri Mantra* has twenty-four syllables and there are twenty-four *Gayatri Mudras* that correspond to the mantra, plus eight additional mudras that are practiced at the conclusion of chanting and meditation.

Twenty-Four Pre-Meditation Mudras

1. Sumukha

2. Samputa

3. Vitita

4. Vistara

5. Dvimukha

6. Trimukha

7. Chaturmukha

8. Panchamukha

9. Shanmukha

10. Adhomukha

11. Vyapak Anjali

12. Shakata

13. Yampasha

14. Granthita

15. Chonmukha Mukha

16. Pralamba

17. Mushtika

18. Matsya

19. Kurma

20. Varaha

21. Simhakranta

22. Mahakranta

23. Mudgara

24. Pallava

Eight Post-Meditation Mudras

1. Surabhi

2. Purna Jnana

3. Vairagya

4. Yoni

5. Shankha

6. Padma

7. Linga

8. Nirvana

APPENDIX C

Dance Mudra Sets

Several established sequences of dance mudras are classified in the *Abhinaya Darpana* and *Natya Shastra*. As an aid to studying these various sets, we have included some of the most common sequences below.

Dashavatara Hastas: Hand Mudras Representing the Ten Incarnations of Vishnu

Dashavatara refers to the ten principal incarnations of *Vishnu* or sometimes *Krishna*. Depicting these ten incarnations and their symbolic hand gestures is a common theme in Classical Indian Dance and other art forms in India. The concept of *Dashavatara* is innermost to *Vaishnavaite* Hinduism, and has deep and encompassing implications on this culture's worldview, spirituality, and art. The *Avatara* doctrine was first clearly articulated in the *Bhagavadgita*, and elaborated upon in the *Puranas, Giga Govinda, Abhinaya Darpana*, and numerous other texts throughout India. It denotes those *avataras* most prominent in terms of their importance in Hindu mythology. The tenth is predicted to appear at the end of the *Kali Yuga*. According to the *Vishnu Purana* and the *Bhagavata Purana*, *Kali Yuga* will end with the apparition of *Kalki Avatara*, who will defeat evil, liberate the virtuous, and initiate a new era.

Sanskrit	English	Primary Mudras	Notes
Matsya	Fish	*Matsya Mudra* held at shoulder level	Moving the hands in a zigzag motion like a swimming fish
Kurma	Tortoise	*Kurma Mudra* held at chest level	Moving the hands back and forth to denote a tortoise
Varaha	Boar	*Varaha Mudra* held at waist level	Moving the hands up and down to denote the charging of a boar

Sanskrit	English	Primary Mudras	Notes
Narasimha	Lion-man	L.H. in *Simhamukha Mudra*. R.H. in *Tripataka Mudra* at chest level	Alternative position is *Ravana Mudra* shaken around the body to denote valor
Vamana	Dwarf	L.H. in an upside-down *Padmakosha Mudra*. R.H. in upside-down *Kapittha Mudra*	L.H. denotes holding an umbrella. R.H. denotes holding a *kamandalu* (an oblong water pot used by ascetics)
Parashurama	Rama-of-the-axe/ Slayer	L.H. is gripping the waist in *Ardhachandra Mudra*. R.H. in *Ardhapataka Mudra* by the shoulder	Alternative position is *Pataka Mudra* denoting the motion of cutting with a battle-axe
Raghurama	*Rama*— Prince of Ayodhya	L.H. in *Sikhara Mudra* held by left shoulder. R.H. in *Katakamukha Mudra III* held by right shoulder	*Rama* is depicted as holding a bow and arrow
Balarama	*Krishna's* elder brother	L.H. in *Sikhara Mudra* and R.H. in *Mushti Mudra,* both held over the left shoulder	*Balarama* is a farmer; these hand positions denote holding the plough
Buddha or *Krishna*	The Enlightened One	*Krishna*: Both hands in *Mrigashirsha Mudra* held above the right shoulder as playing a flute. *Buddha*: Both hands in *Dola Mudra* by the two sides	This *avatara* differs between the texts. In the *Abhinaya Darpana*, it is noted as *Krishna*. According to the *Gita Govinda*, it is *Buddha*
Kali	"Eternity," or Destroyer of evil	R.H. in *Pataka Mudra* above the head facing leftward. L.H. in *Tripataka Mudra* pointing forward at waist level	*Kalki* is depicted riding a white horse with a blazing sword and is anticipated to appear in the end of *Kali Yuga* to terminate evil and bring in the age of kindness

Varna Hastas: Hand Mudras Denoting the Four Castes

Sanskrit	English	Left Hand	Right Hand	Notes
Brahmana	*Brahmin*, the priestly caste of Hindu society	*Shikhara* held above left shoulder with the thumb facing downward	Form *Sikhara*, and move the tip of the thumb from the left shoulder obliquely to the right hip	This Mudra symbolizes the sacred thread which is the mark of a *Brahmin*
Kshatriya	"Warrior"—this caste is primarily comprised of leaders	*Shikhara*, moves obliquely across the body	*Pataka* held by the right shoulder and faces outward	
Vaishya	This caste primarily comprises of merchants, farmers, and artists	*Hamsasya* facing outward	*Katakamukha I* facing outward	
Shudra	The "servants" caste, comprises of service jobs	*Shikhara* held in front of chest	*Suchi* held by right shoulder	

Ashta Digpala Hastas: Hand Mudras Representing the Guardians of the Eight Directions

The Guardians of the Directions are the deities who rule the specific directions of space according to Hinduism and *Vajrayana* Buddhism. As a group of eight deities, they are called *Ashta Digpala*, literally meaning guardians of eight directions. They are often augmented with two extra deities for the ten directions (the two extra directions being zenith and nadir), when they are known as the *Dasha Digpala*.

Name	Direction	Hands	Weapon	Consort	Matrika
Kubera	North	R: Mushti L: Alapadma	Gada (mace)	Kuberajaya	Kumari
Yama	South	R: Suchi L: Tamrachuda	Danda (staff)	Yami	Varahi
Indra	East	Two Tripataka crossed	Vajra (thunderbolt)	Sachi	Aindri
Varuna	West	R: Pataka L: Shikhara	Pasa (noose)	Nalani	Varuni
Ishana	Northeast	R: Tripataka L: Mushti crossed	Trishula (trident)	Parvati	Maheshvari
Agni	Southeast	R: Tripataka L: Kangula	Shakti (spear)	Svaha	Meshavahini
Vayu	Northeast	R: Arala L: Ardhapataka	Ankusha (goad)	Bharati	Mrigavahini
Nirriti	Southwest	R: Shakata L: Katva	Khadga (sword)	Khadgi	Khadagadhari
Vishnu (extra)	Nadir	Tripataka with both hands	Chakra (discus)	Lakshmi	Vaishnavi
Brahma (extra)	Zenith	R: Hamsasya L: Chatura	Padma (lotus)	Sarasvati	Brahmani

Deva Hastas: Hand Mudras Representing the Sixteen Gods and Goddesses

Name	Right Hand	Left Hand
Brahma	*Hamsasya*	*Chatura*
Vishnu	*Tripataka*	*Tripataka*
Shiva	*Tripataka*	*Mrigashirsha*
Sarasvati	*Suchi*	*Kapittha*
Lakshmi	*Kapittha*	*Kapittha*
Parvati	*Ardhachandra*	*Ardhachandra*
Vighneshvara	*Kapittha*	*Kapittha*
Shanmukha	*Shikhara*	*Trishula*
Manmatha	*Katakamukha*	*Shikhara*
Indra	*Tripataka*	*Tripataka*
Varuna	*Pataka*	*Shikhara*
Vayu	*Arala*	*Ardhapataka*
Agni	*Tripataka*	*Kangula*
Kubera	*Mushti*	*Alapadma*
Nirriti	*Shakata*	*Katva*
Yama	*Suchi*	*Tamrachuda*

Navagraha Hasta: Hand Mudras
Representing the Nine Planets

Sanskrit	English	Right Hand	Left Hand
Surya	Sun	*Kapittha*	*Alapadma*
Chandra	Moon	*Pataka*	*Alapadma*
Angaraka	Mars	*Mushti*	*Suchi*
Budha	Mercury	*Pataka*	*Shikhara* or *Mushti*
Guru	Jupiter	*Shikhara*	*Shikhara*
Shukra	Venus	*Mushti*	*Mushti*
Shani	Saturn	*Trishula*	*Shikhara*
Rahu	"South node"	*Suchi*	*Sarpashirsha*
Ketu	"North node"	*Pataka*	*Suchi*

Bandhava Hastas: Hand Mudras
Representing the Eleven Relationships

Sanskrit	English	Right Hand	Left Hand	Notes
Dampati	Husband and wife	*Mrigashirsha*	*Shikhara*	Indicating female (right) and male (left)
Matri	Mother/Daughter	*Samdamsa*	*Ardhachandra*	Left hand placed on abdomen indicates women or womb
Pitri	Father	*Shikhara*	*Samdamsa*	
Shvashru	Mother-in-law	*Hamsasya*	*Ardhachandra*	Left hand placed on abdomen indicates women or womb
Shvashura	Father-in-law	*Shikhara*	*Hamsasya*	
Bhartri Bhratri	Brother-in-law	*Kartarimukha*	*Shikhara*	

Nanandri	Sister-in-law	*Kartarimukha* or *Shikhara*	*Mrigashirsha*	Left hand placed on abdomen indicates women or womb
Jyeshtha Kanishtha Bhratri	Elder or younger brother	*Mayura*	*Shikhara*	Move the hands back and forth alternately
Snusha	Daughter-in-law	*Mrigashirsha*	*Mayura*	Right hand placed on abdomen indicates women or womb
Bhartri	Husband	*Shikhara*	*Hamsasya*	Held by the throat
Sapatni	Co-wife	*Pasha to Mrigashirsha*	*Pasha to Mrigashirsha*	Place *Mrigashirsha* hands on abdomen to indicate women or womb

The Twenty-eight *Samyukta Hastas* (Single-Hand Mudras)

1. *Pataka*—"flag"

2. *Tripataka*—"three parts of the flag"

3. *Ardhapataka*—"half-flag"

4. *Kartarimukha*—"arrow face"

5. *Mayura*—"peacock"

6. *Ardhachandra*—"half-moon"

7. *Arala*—"bent" or "crooked"

8. *Shukatunda*—"parrot's beak"

9. *Mushti*—"fist"

10. *Shikhara*—"spire" or "peak of the mountain"

11. *Kapittha*—"elephant apple" or "wood apple"

12. *Katakamukha*—"link in a chain"

13. *Suchi*—"needle"

14. *Chandrakala*—"crescent moon"

15. *Padmakosha*—"lotus bud"

16. *Sarpashirsha*—"serpent head"

17. *Mrigashirsha*—"deer head"

18. *Simhamukha*—"lion face"

19. *Kangula*—"tail" or "plough" or "hand"

20. *Alapadma*—"fully opened lotus"

21. *Chatura*—"jackal" or "clever"

22. *Bhramara*—"bee"

23. *Hamsasya*—"swan's face"

24. *Hamsapaksha*—"swan's wing"

25. *Samdamsha*—"grasping"

26. *Mukula*—"bud"

27. *Tamrachuda*—"rooster"

28. *Trishula*—"trident"

The Twenty-four *Asamyukta Hastas* (Joint-Hand Mudras)

1. *Anjali*—"prayer" or "salutation"

2. *Kapota*—"dove"

3. *Karkata*—"crab"

4. *Svastika*—"crossed"

5. *Dola*—"swing"

6. *Pushpaputa*—"flower-casket"

7. *Utsanga*—"embrace"

8. *Shivalinga*—"masculine creative energy"

9. *Katakavardhana*—"link of increase"

10. *Kartarisvastika*—"crossed arrows"

11. *Shakata*—"cart" or "carriage"

12. *Shankha*—"conch shell"

13. *Chakra*—"wheel" or "discus"

14. *Samputa*—"casket"

15. *Pasha*—"noose"

16. *Kilaka*—"bond"

17. *Matsya*—"fish"

18. *Kurma*—"tortoise"

19. *Varaha*—"boar"

20. *Garuda*—"mythological bird"

21. *Nagabandha*—"serpent tie"

22. *Khatva*—"cot"

23. *Bherunda*—"pair of birds" or "two-headed bird"

24. *Avahita*—"dissimulation" or "holding things"

Endnotes

Introduction

1   Literally, *yoga* ("union"), *tattva* ("principle/element"), *mudra* ("hand position"), *vijnana* ("science" or "knowledge")—the science and discipline of maintaining harmony by using finger positions related to the elements.

2   One of the most important texts of the Kaula School of Tantrism.

3   Literally ("the fourth"), meaning the realm of Immediate Presence beyond the normal three states of being: waking, sleeping, and dreaming.

4   *Kanaphata* ("ear split") refers to the large earrings they wear. They are sometimes referred to as Tantric *sannyasins* (ascetics), because of their emphasis in acquiring *siddhis* (supernatural powers) in contrast to more orthodox practices of purification, devotion, and meditation.

5   See: Dor-je, Wan-ch'ug. *The Mahamudra: Eliminating the Darkness of Ignorance.* New Delhi, India: Library of Tibetan Works and Archives, 1978.

6   Such as *Ashvini Mudra, Bhujangini Mudra, Khecari Mudra, Maha Mudra, Manduki Mudra, Matangi Mudra, Sahajoli Mudra, Shakticalani Mudra, Shambhavi Mudra, Vajroli Mudra, Yoni Mudra*, and so forth.

7   Literally ("first lord"), another name for *Shiva*.

8   See: Muktibodhananda, Swami, trans. *Hatha Yoga Pradipika: Light on Hatha Yoga.* Bihar, India: Bihar School of Yoga, 1993, pp.286–290.

9   Satchidananda, Swami. *Integral Yoga Hatha.* New York: Hold, Rinehart and Winston, 1970, p.156.

10   See: Apparao, P.S.R., trans. *Abhinaya Darpanam of Nandikeswara.* Hyderabad, India: Natyamala Publications, 1997, p.44.

11   See: Iyengar, B.K.S. *Light on Yoga.* New York: Stockton Books, 1979, p.131.

12   See: Iyengar, B.K.S. *Light on Yoga.* New York: Stockton Books, 1979, p.120.

The Mudras

1   Synonymous with the idea of Original Nature.

2   Earth, Water, Fire, Air, and Ether.

3   A treatise on dance from Kerala that informs the usage of hand gestures in *Katahkhali* and *Mohiniyattam* dance.

4   "Lord of the farmland," a deity who was originally considered the local spirit of the farmland, particularly in southern India. His image is generally placed on the

northeastern corner of temples devoted to *Shiva*, and he is worshipped prior to each ritual to ensure efficacy.

5   "Mover of mountains," a famous sage revered in southern India. He is said to have introduced the Vedic tradition and was instrumental in the formation of language and literature.

6   "Good," "beneficial," or "divine (being)," an ancient god of western India. Also known as *Krishna*'s father. Sometimes used synonymously with the name *Krishna*.

7   A short treatise on Odissi Dance allegedly completed in 1670.

8   The seven accoutrements a universal monarch must possess to stay in power: the precious queen, the precious general, the precious horse, the precious jewel, the precious minister, the precious elephant, and the precious wheel.

9   A sage and devotee of *Vishnu*. According to legend, his devotion was so strong that it moved *Vishnu* to save him during the great flood.

10 "Unlimited," "free," or "unbounded," the Vedic goddess of space (*Kasha*), the mother of all creatures and gods.

11 See: Apparao, P.S.R., trans. *Abhinaya Darpanam of Nandikeswara.* Hyderabad, India: Natyamala Publications, 1997, p.392.

12 An emanation of *Shiva* from southern India emphasizing his dancing form. His right leg is firmly placed on the personification of *apasmarapurusha* (ignorance), and his left leg is raised halfway into the air as he begins to dance.

13 Aspect of the *Devi*, and one of the *Saptamatrikas* (eight matriarchs). Generally represented as a woman with a boar's head.

14 A short Sanskrit text epitomizing the non-dual teachings of *Advaita Vedanta*.

15 The absolute soul or supreme spirit concept in Vedanta and Yoga philosophies.

16 An ancient Indian stringed instrument that the goddess *Sarasvati* is often depicted playing.

17 "The south-facing image of *Shiva*"—the aspect of *Shiva* as the ultimate ascetic and quintessential guru of music, philosophy, and yoga.

18 Literally "reality," or "principles of reality." Traditionally, the *Samkya* system of philosophy recognizes twenty-four *tattvas*; such as *buddhi* (higher mind), *manas* (lower mind), *indriya* (senses), and so forth.

19 The sound and vibration of Om. Meditation on Om, as the primal sound of creation, is a technique described in numerous Sanskrit texts on yoga, such as the *Bhagavad Gita, Upanishads,* and *Yoga Sutras of Patanjali.*

20 Pure Dance, lyrical variations of a musical raga.

21 See: Odissi Research Centre. *Odissi Dance Pathfinder Vol. I.* Bhubaneswar, India: Smt. Kum Kum Mohanty, 1998, p.42.

22 A prominent sage from ancient times referred to as "Old Tortoise Man," considered to be the ancestral father of the *devas, asuras, nagas,* and human beings.

23 Another name for *Kartikeya*, the son of *Shiva*, and the commander of the army of the gods.

24 See: Odissi Research Centre. *Odissi Dance Pathfinder Vol. I.* Bhubaneswar, India: Smt. Kum Kum Mohanty, 1998, p.43.

25 Alternative name for *Kubera*, the god of wealth. Represented as "the king of nature-spirits."

26 In the Tantric tradition, *Shiva* represents intrinsic clarity, pristine awareness, unborn, unchanging, unswerving acceptance. *Shakti* represents primal creativity, birth, life, and death, limitless manifestations, and constantly change.

27 A king who had attained heaven.

28 Originally commissioned by Emperor Ashoka in the third century BCE to contain relics of the historical Buddha, and as an emblem of his newly aroused affection for Buddhism. It is considered one of the oldest stone temple structures in India.

29 The mythological center of the universe, located in the Himalayan mountains (in modern Tibet), believed to be the abode of *Shiva*. Also called the Golden Mountain.

30 A mark on the forehead representing the "third eye," or the idea of spiritual vision. Usually made with sandalwood paste, sindhur, or ashes (*vibhuti*) from the sacred fire.

31 "Brilliant," "golden," or "yellow"—synonymous with *Parvati*, consort of *Shiva*. She is reputed as the embodiment of motherhood.

32 Ascetic spiritual discipline.

33 Mentioned in the *Shiva Samhita, Hatha Yoga Pradipika*, and *Yoga Yajnyavalaya*, *kanda* literally means "bulb," and is the name given to the energetic structure in the lower abdomen considered to be the origin of the *nadis* (energy channels).

34 A *naga* (snake) that takes human birth through *Devaki*, one of the primal beings of creation. In the *Puranas, Shesha* is said to hold all the planets of the universe on his hoods and to constantly sing of the glory of *Vishnu* from all his mouths.

35 Musician to the gods, lead singer of the *Gandharvas* (celestial musicians).

36 Literally "worship of the limbs of the body," a ritual practice of remembering the preciousness of human life and the sacredness of the human body.

37 A revered Vedic *siddha* (adept) credited with uncovering many of the mantras of the *Rig Veda*.

38 As performed in the *arti* ritual, where the Five Elements (in the form of fire, incense, flowers, peacock fan, and yak-tail whisk) are offered in devotion to the Divine.

39 *Sarasvati*: literally *saras*, "flow," and *vati*, "woman." The unfolding of knowledge is likened to a flowing river that nourishes those who seek it. To those who desire knowledge it is said to be supremely alluring, like a beautiful woman.

40 The powerful king of the *asuras* (demons).

41 Another name for the deity *Kartikeya*, who was born from *Shiva's* concentration as a spark of fire from his "third eye."

42 See Note 30.

43 In the context of Hindu mythology it is believed to be a cosmic column. The *stambha* symbolizes the bond which joins heaven and earth. A number of Hindu scriptures, including the *Atharva Veda*, have references to *stambha*.

44 "All-maker," the architect of the universe, *Vishvakarma* represents the supreme creative power, knowledge, and wisdom.

45 See: Apparao, P.S.R., trans. *Abhinaya Darpanam of Nandikeswara.* Hyderabad, India: Natyamala Publications, 1997, p.391.

46 See note 23.

47 The incarnation of *Vishnu* as a tortoise.

48 He is the great king of the *nagas* ("mythological serpent") who wears a gem (*nagamani*) on his head.

49 For example, *Narasimha* is described as using his hands to tear the *raksasa's* (demon) chest in a fierce battle to protect devotees from evil.

50 Alternate nostril breathing.

51 There are numerous subtleties to this application of *Vishnu Mudra* that are too complex to explain here. Such nuances are best learned from a competent teacher of yoga and pranayama.

Appendix A

1 For information on traditional chakra colors, see: Avalon, Arthur. *The Serpent Power: The secrets of Tantric and Shaktic Yoga.* Madras, India: Dover Publications, 1974.

GLOSSARY

ABHINAYA ("lead toward") The concept in Indian dance and drama referring to the art of dramatic expression. Etymologically it is derived from the Sanskrit *abhi* ("toward") and *nii* ("leading/guide"), literally meaning "to lead toward," as in leading the audience toward a particular sentiment. *Abhinaya* is an integral part of all the Indian Classical Dance styles, where hand mudras as well as facial expression are heavily utilized as instruments of story telling.

ABHINAYA CHANDRIKA A regional treatise on dance written by Maheshvara Mohapatra circa 1670 CE. It includes a detailed description of the various movements of the feet and hands, as well as the postures and movements unique to the region of modern-day Orissa.

ABHINAYA DARPANA A treatise written in third or fourth century CE by Nandikeshvara. This text's main focus is the techniques of communication in dance, and is widely followed by South Indian dance forms.

ADVAITA VEDANTA ("non-dual Vedanta") One of India's most influential philosophical systems.

AGNI ("fire") One of the *pancha mahabhuta*, "five elemental principles," of the Indian cosmological system.

AJNA CHAKRA ("command center") The energy center located between the eyebrows, commonly called the "third eye," related to the pineal gland.

AKASHA ("space") One of the *pancha mahabhuta*, "five elemental principles," of the Indian cosmological system.

ANAHATA CHAKRA ("un-struck sound") The energy center located behind the heart, at the center of the chest, related to the cardiac plexus and the thymus gland.

ANGIKABHINAYA ("physical expression") The usage of hand mudras in Indian dance and drama to convey an elaborate repertoire of meaning.

APANA ("downward moving force") Refers to *apana vayu*, one of the Five Vital Winds (*pancha vayu*) inside the human body.

ASHTAVAKRAGITA ("song of Ashtavakra") A short Sanskrit text epitomizing the non-dual teachings of *Advaita Vedanta*.

ASURA ("unwise deity") A class of beings (lesser deities) in Hindu cosmology characterized by greed, jealousy, paranoia, and constant quarreling.

AYURVEDA ("science of life") *Ayu* ("longevity"), *veda* ("knowledge"); the traditional system of holistic medicine native to India.

BHAVA ("sentiment") Status of being, a subjective becoming, states of mind; from the Sanskrit *bhu* ("to become"). Most frequently translated as feeling, emotion, mood, and devotional state.

BINDU ("point" or "drop") The central point of focus in a geometric figure, a point of concentration, a drop of semen representing the primal creative force.

DEDICATE THE MERIT The ritual of sharing the benefit of one's practice with all beings. In Buddhist and yogic traditions, this is traditionally included at the conclusion of every practice session.

DEVA ("celestial" or "shining") A class of benevolent supernatural beings, or gods in the Hindu pantheon; sometimes called nature spirits.

DURGA ("inaccessible") One of the many aspects of Devi (the divine feminine principal), the creator and destroyer of humanity and nature, known as a fierce warrior against enemies of the *Dharma*, she is considered matriarch of the sixty-four yoginis.

EARTH ELEMENT ("*prithvi*") One of the *pancha mahabhuta*, "five elemental principles," used in Indian cosmology to describe the densest of elements.

ETHER ELEMENT ("*akasha*") One of the *pancha mahabhuta*, "five elemental principles," of the Indian cosmological system employed by yoga and Ayurveda used to describe the lightest of elements.

FIRE ELEMENT ("*agni*") One of the *pancha mahabhuta*, "five elemental principles," associated with heat and brightness, internally with digestion and the power to transform.

GREAT STUPA AT SANCHI A sacred Buddhist historical site located in the Indian state of Madhya Pradesh.

GYATRI MANTRA A poetic Sanskrit verse from the Rig Veda consisting of twenty-four syllables, addressing the Sun (*Savitar*). Used as a mantra, this famous verse is chanted morning and evening by millions of people each day.

HASTA ("hand") Relating to the hand or hands. Hasta is also a synonym for hand mudra in the dance tradition, and is the preferred term among scholars to describe the many hand gestures of Indian dance.

JALA ("water") One of the *pancha mahabhuta*, "five elemental principles," of the Indian cosmological system.

KALI ("dark") Perhaps the most famous goddess of the Indian pantheon, depicted as dark-skinned, naked, and ferocious, all traits that hint at the dissolution of all things into the vastness of time and space; the consort of Lord Shiva, personifying both the creative and destructive forces of nature.

KI ("vital force") The Japanese term for "vital energy," similar to *prana* in Sanskrit.

LASYA ("feminine dance") According to Indian mythology, *lasya* describes a graceful and sensual dance originally performed by the goddess Parvati in response to the primal male energy created by Lord Shiva's Tandava dance.

LINGA ("generative organ") The most common symbol associated with Shiva, usually made from an erect stone (loosely resembling a phallus), that represents the creative forces supporting all creation, the beginning and end of the manifest world, usually depicted as *linga* and *yoni* together, symbolizing the manifest and unmanifest aspects of reality.

MANDALA ("circular" or "heavenly orbit") A concentric diagram or cosmological chart used in Hindu and Buddhist ritual as a visual representation of a specific spiritual state, realm, or deity. Often used by practitioners as an object of contemplation designed to take the mind into progressively deeper states of absorption.

MANIPURA CHAKRA ("city of jewels") The energy center located behind the navel, related to the solar plexus and adrenal glands.

MOUNT MERU The mythological center of the universe, the Golden Mountain, located in the Himalayan mountains (in modern Tibet), believed to be the abode of Shiva.

NAGA ("serpent") Most commonly a cobra, a term used in Hindu, Buddhist, and Jain legends to describe a class of semi-divine beings that are half-human and half-serpent, highly intelligent, beautiful, and possessing super-human powers. They are said to dwell in underwater caves and are the guardians of precious metals, gems, and other riches of the earth.

NATYA ("dance" or "performance") A term denoting "drama," includes expressive dance as a key component. Rhythm and lyrical elements preponderate traditional Hindu plays.

NATYA SHASTRA Ascribed to Bharata Muni, and considered the original available treatise on the arts of music, dance, and theatre. It is generally agreed upon to have been written between 200 BCE and 200 CE.

NRITTA ("pure dance") Technical movement within specific rhythm patterns of Indian dance.

NRITYA The dramatic miming aspect of India dance. Also referred to as *Abhinaya* or *Angikabhinaya*.

OJAS ("vitality") The term used in Ayurveda and yoga to describe the storehouse of vigor in the human body, commonly called "the fluid of life."

OM The primordial sound of creation, the seed mantra from which all other mantras originate.

OPENNESS A term used to denote the quality of total acceptance, and the insight of the self-resolving nature of all phenomena; a synonym for Original Nature.

PALLAVI ("pure dance") Lyrical variations of a musical raga.

PERINEUM The diamond shaped region of the human body located between the pubic symphysis and the coccyx, inferior to the pelvic diaphragm.

PRANA ("vital breath" or "life-force") Generally used to denote the basic energy of the universe. Specifically used in the yogic system to describe one of the Five Vayus; *Prana Vayu* is the energy located in the region of the chest and is associated with the heart and lungs.

PRANAYAMA ("breath control") The elaborate system of breathing exercises employed in yoga to induce various internal states and affect the nervous, endocrine, circulatory, and respiratory systems.

PRATYAHARA ("interiorization of the senses") One of the limbs of the Eight-Fold Path of yoga, where the aspirant reduces their attachment to sensory stimuli in an effort to lead the mind into subtler states of mediation.

PRAYOGA ("proper action") Denotes the "right" way of applying any art or action.

PRITHIVI ("earth") One of the *pancha mahabhuta*, "five elemental principles," of the Indian cosmological system.

PUJA ("worship") The performance specific ritual for a deity, aspect of nature, or guru.

QI ("fragrant steam") The Chinese word for life-force, poetically symbolized by the aromatic steam rising from freshly cooked rice. The energy animating the universe and flowing within the human body, similar to *prana* in Sanskrit, or *ki* in Japanese.

RASA ("juice" or "essence") Generally refers to the inner emotional experience created by *bhavas*.

SAHASRARA CHAKRA ("thousand-petalled lotus") The energy center located at the crown of the head, related to the pituitary gland and hypothalamus.

SHAKAMUNI BUDDHA The historical Buddha, Siddhartha Gautama, a spiritual teacher from ancient India (the region is now within the borders of modern Nepal), upon whose teachings Buddhism is founded.

SHAVASANA ("corpse pose") The reclining rest posture commonly used in Hatha Yoga at the conclusion of a series of *asanas* (postures).

SHIVA ("benign") The Hindu deity of Absolute Reality, model of the perfect yogi.

SOLAR PLEXUS A complex network of nerves located behind the stomach.

SUSHUMNA NADI ("central channel") The energy pathway containing the seven chakras of the Indian Tantric tradition, that runs through the center of the spine, from the pelvic floor to the top of the head.

SVADHISTHANA CHAKRA ("one's own abode") The energy center located behind the pubic bone, associated with the coccyx, testes, and ovaries.

TANTRA ("net" or "loom") The spiritual path of ritual and transformation, emphasizing worship of feminine principal (*Shakti*), employs a wide range of diverse methods to awaken the latent potential of body, mind, and spirit.

TANTRIC BUDDHISM ("*Vajrayana*") One of the traditional vehicles of Buddhist practice.

TEJAS ("brightness") According to the traditions of yoga and Ayurveda, *tejas* is the force of transformation within the body/mind of the individual, responsible for mental clarity, digestion, assimilation, motivation, regulating body heat, etc.

VAHANA ("vehicle") Describes the animal or mythological creature a *deva* uses for transportation.

VAJRASANA ("thunderbolt pose") A traditional posture used in Hatha Yoga to improve digestion and increase suppleness in the lower body. Performed by kneeling with the inner thighs together and the buttocks resting lightly on the heels.

VAJRAYANA ("diamond vehicle") The path of Tantric Buddhism.

VASUDEVA ("supreme being") The father of Krishna, and also used as an alternate name for Krishna himself.

VAYU ("air") One of the *pancha mahabhuta*, "five elemental principles," of the Indian cosmological system.

VINIYOGA ("right application") The traditional dance and theatre usages of hand gestures described in the *Abhinaya Darpana* and the *Natya Shastra*.

VISHNU ("preserver") The Hindu deity worshiped in many forms or incarnations (*avataras*), the two most common being Rama and Krishna.

VISHUDDHA CHAKRA ("wheel of nectar") The energy center located in the pit of the throat, associated with the thyroid gland, pharynx, and larynx.

WATER ELEMENT ("*jala*") One of the *pancha mahabhuta*, "five elemental principles," of the Indian cosmological system.

YAJNA ("sacrifice") The practice of ritual offering central to Hindu religion.

YANTRA ("instrument") A geometric symbol used for visualization and meditation usually representing the manifestation of a specific deity or spiritual realm.

YOGA TATTVA MUDRA VIJNANA A branch of yogic knowledge used for healing and spiritual cultivation that deals with the relationship between the five fingers and Five Elements (*pancha mahabhuta*), and how to employ this knowledge to form hand gestures to create specific desired effects.

YONI ("source" or "vagina") The symbol of the divine feminine principle, and the source of all creation.

BIBLIOGRAPHY

Akers, Brian Dana, trans. *The Hatha Yoga Pradipika*. Woodstock, NY: Yoga Vidya, 2002.

Apparao, P.S.R., trans. *Abhinaya Darpanam of Nandikeswara*. Hyderabad, India: Natyamala Publications, 1997.

Avalon, Arthur. *The Serpent Power: The secrets of Tantric and Shaktic Yoga*. Madras, India: Dover Publications, 1974.

Bansal, Vijay K. *Good Health Without Medicines*. Gaziabad, India: Vijay K. Bansal, 2008.

Bharatamuni, trans. by a board of scholars. *The Natya Shastra*. Delhi, India: Sri Satguru Publications, 1986–2003.

Bose, Mandakranta. *The Dance Vocabulary of Classical India*. Delhi, India: Sri Satguru Publications, 1995.

Bunce, Fredrick W. *Mudras in Buddhist and Hindu Practices: An Iconographical Consideration*. New Delhi, India: D.K. Printworld, 2001.

Byrom, Thomas, trans. *The Heart of Awareness: A Translation of the Ashtavakra Gita*. Boston, MA: Shambhala Publications, 1990.

Coomaraswamy, Ananda and Duggirala, Gopala Kristnayya, trans. *The Mirror of Gesture*. London: Humphrey Milford, 1917.

Dallapiccola, Anna L. *Dictionary of Hindu Lore and Legend*. London: Thames & Hudson, 2002.

Devi, Nischala Joy. *The Healing Path of Yoga*. New York, NY: Three Rivers Press, 2000.

Dor-je, Wan-ch'ug. *The Mahamudra: Eliminating the Darkness of Ignorance*. New Delhi, India: Library of Tibetan Works and Archives, 1978.

Feuerstein, Georg. *The Yoga Tradition: Its History, Literature, Philosophy and Practice*. Prescott, AZ: Hohm Press, 2001.

Feuerstein, Georg. *The Shambhala Encyclopedia of Yoga*. Boston, MA: Shambhala Publications, 1997.

Gharote, M.L. and Devnath, Parimal, eds. *Hathapradipika of Svatmarama*. Bhangarwadi, India: Lonavla Yoga Institute, 2001.

Ghosh, Manomohan. *Nandikesvara Abhinayadarpanam*. Calcutta, India: Manisha, 2006.

Govindarajan, Hema. *The Nrtyavinoda of Manasollasa, a Study*. New Delhi, India: Harman Publishing House, 2001.

Hirschi, Gertrud. *Mudras: Yoga in Your Hands*. York Beach, ME: Samuel Weiser, 2000.

Iyengar, B.K.S. *Light on Yoga*. New York: Stockton Books, 1979.

Jansen, Eva Rudy. *The Book of Hindu Imagery*. New Delhi, India: New Age Books, 2005.

Keshav Dev, Acharya. *Mudras for Healing*. New Delhi, India: Aacharya Shri Enterprises, 1995.

Keshav Dev, Acharya. *Healing Hands: Science of Yoga Mudras*. New Delhi, India: Aacharya Shri Enterprises, 2008.

Londhe, Veena and Agneswaran, Malati. *Hand Book of Indian Classical Dance Terminology*. Bombay, India: Nalanda Dance Research Centre, 1992.

Mallinson, James, trans. *The Shiva Samhita*. Woodstock, NY: Yoga Vidya, 2007.

Mallinson, James, trans. *The Gheranda Samhita*. Woodstock, NY: Yoga Vidya, 2004.

Menen, Rajendar. *The Healing Power of Mudras*. Delhi, India: Pustak Mahal, 2009.

Mohapatra, Maheswar. *Abhinaya Chandrika*, trans. by Pattnaik, Dhirendra Nath. Cuttack, Orissa, India: Kala Vikash Kendra Trust Board, 1999.

Mookerjee, Ajit. *Kali: The Feminine Force*. London: Thames & Hudson, 1998.

Mookerjee, Ajit. *Kundalini: The Arousal of Inner Energy*. London: Thames & Hudson, 1982.

Mohan, A.G., trans. *Yoga-Yajnavalkya*. Madras, India: Ganesh & Co., 2000.

Muktibodhananda, Swami, trans. *Hatha Yoga Pradipika: Light on Hatha Yoga*. Bihar, India: Bihar School of Yoga, 1993.

Muni, Swami Rajarshi. *Yoga: The Ultimate Spiritual Path*. St. Paul, MN: Llewellyn Publications, 2001.

Neog, Maheswar. *Srihastamuktavali*. New Delhi, India: Indira Gandhi National Centre for the Arts, 1991.

Nivedita, Sister and Coomaraswamy, Ananda. *Myths and Legends of the Hindus and Buddhists*. Kolkata, India: Advaita Ashrama, 2001.

Odissi Research Centre. *Odissi Dance Path Finder Vol. I and II*. Bhubaneswar, India: Smt. Kum Kum Mohanty, 1998.

Raut, Madhumita. *Odissi What, Why and How: Evolution, Revival and Technique*. Delhi, India: BR Rhythms Publication, 2007.

Saraswati, Swami Satyananda. *Asana Pranayama Mudra Bandha*. Bihar, India: Yoga Publications Trust, 1996.

Satchidananda, Swami. *Integral Yoga Hatha*. New York, NY: Holt, Rinehart and Winston, 1970.

Singh, Jaideva, trans. *Pratyabhijnahrdayam: The Secret of Self-Recognition*. Delhi, India: Motilal Banarsidass Publishers, 2011.

Singh, Jaideva, trans. *Siva Sutras: The Yoga of Supreme Identity*. Delhi, India: Motilal Banarsidass Publishers, 2008.

Singh, Jaideva, trans. *Spanda-Karikas: The Divine Creative Pulsation*. Delhi, India: Motilal Banarsidass Publishers, 2007.

Trungpa, Chogyam. *Mudra: Early Poems and Songs*. Boston, MA: Shambhala, 1972.

Vatsyayan, Kapila. *Indian Classical Dance*. New Delhi, India: Ministry of Information and Broadcasting Government of India, 1974.

Werner, Karel. *A Popular Dictionary of Hinduism*. Chicago, IL: NTC Publishing Group, 1997.

Williams, Emily Fuller. *Mudras: Ancient Gestures to Ease Modern Stress*. Seattle, WA: Parenting Press, 2011.

Wu, Zhongxian. *Vital Breath of the Dao: Chinese Shamanic Tiger Qigong*. St. Paul, MN: Dragon Door Publications, 2006.

Zimmer, Heinrich. *Myths and Symbols in Indian Art and Civilization*. Princeton, NJ: Princeton University Press, 1992.

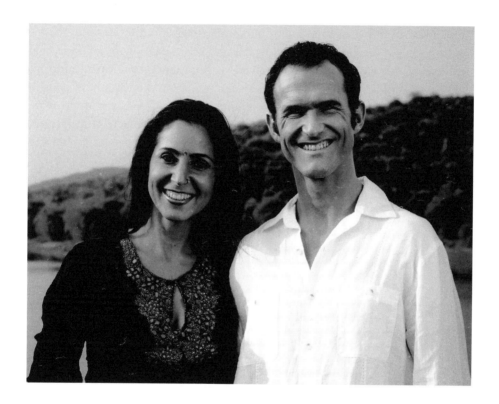

Cain Carroll

Cain Carroll teaches yoga, qigong, meditation, and self-healing worldwide. He has trained extensively under the guidance of Daoist, Buddhist, and Indian yoga masters. His journeys have taken him to remote areas of India, China, Nepal, Tibet, Thailand, and South America, where he received private instruction in numerous systems of practice. Cain is co-author of *Partner Yoga: Making Contact for Physical, Emotional and Spiritual Growth* (Rodale 2000) and creator of three self-healing DVDs: *Pain-Free Joints*, *Heal Neck and Shoulder Pain*, and *Digestive Power*. He served for two years as the Director of Yoga Teacher Training at Southwest Institute of Healing Arts (Tempe, AZ), and four years as Yoga Director and co-owner of Yoga Shala (Prescott, AZ). Please visit www.caincarroll.com for more information.

Revital Carroll

Native to the land of Israel, Revital has been dedicated to the study of Indian spiritual arts since childhood. Intensive study and practice of yoga and meditation in the Himalayas led her to discover her passion for Indian dance where she finds the sensual and the spiritual expressing as one. She is the creator of three instructional DVDs: *Temple Goddess Workout*, *Odissi Dance Foundations*, and *Odissi Dance Spins and Choreography*, and her articles about Classical Indian Dance and yoga appeared in numerous magazines. Revital offers classes, workshops and performances worldwide. She was the co-owner of Yoga Shala in Prescott, AZ, and the director of several yoga programs in North California. She draws her inspiration from the elements of nature, the wisdom of her own body, and the rich spiritual heritage of ancient India. She currently lives and teaches in the bay area of San Francisco. Visit www.shaktibhakti.com for more information.

INDEX